Carb
Cycling

A Doable and Once and for All Solution to Losing Weight

(Recipes and Exercises to Unlocking the Power and Build Muscle)

Ronald Hogue

Published By **Bella Frost**

Ronald Hogue

Carb Cycling: A Doable and Once and for All Solution to Losing Weight (Recipes and Exercises to Unlocking the Power and Build Muscle)

ISBN   978-1-998769-15-5

No part of this guidebook shall be reproduced in any form without permission in writing from the publisher except in the case of brief quotations embodied in critical articles or reviews.

Legal & Disclaimer

Table Of Contents

Chapter 1: What Is Carb Cycling And How Do You Get It?.. 1

Chapter 2: The Theory Behind Carbcycling................. 8

Chapter 3: How Carb Cycling Works...........................15

Chapter 4: Carb Cycling Facts And Fatloss.................20

Chapter 5: Advanced Fat Loss, And Why Carb Cycling Works...24

Chapter 6: Breaking Through The Diet Plateau..........29

Chapter 7: Carb Cycling To Help You Lose Weight.....35

Chapter 8: Frequently Asked Questions.....................41

Chapter 9: Get Started! 48

Chapter 10: A 4 Week Carb Cycling Meal Plan...........54

Chapter 11: The Origin Of Carb Cycling & The Low Carb Diet 63

Chapter 12: The Fundamental Principles Of Carb Cycling...68

Chapter 13: Carbohydrate Patterning 71

Chapter 14: The Nuances Of Carb Cycling 79

Chapter 15: Getting Past The Fat Burning Plateau.....87

Chapter 16: Sample Meal Plans For Carb Cycling.......90

BREAKFAST RECIPES 117

Mango Coconut Yogurt Bowl 117

Apple Pie Overnight Oats..118

Low Carb Creamy Egg Cups with Bacon & Egg.........119

Keto Sausage Balls Recipe, Low Carb 121

Oven-Baked Easter Eggs in A Muffin Tin.................123

Sausage Egg Muffins...124

90-Second Keto French Toast 126

Keto Low Carb Bagels Recipe Using Fathead Dough
Gluten Free 128

Herb Baked Eggs...129

Keto Berry Mug Cake...131

Keto Blueberry Pancakes Gluten-Free....................132

Low Carb Pumpkin waffles......................................134

Baked Tomato Eggs 137

Baked Eggs In Avocado 138

Chicken And Apple Sausage....................................140

Baked Eggs in Ham Cups..141

Mexican Breakfast Bowl 143

LUNCH RECIPES 144

Avocado Bacon Crustless Quiche Recipe.................144

Buffalo Chicken and Broccoli Bowls 145

Grilled Salmon Kebabs...148

Healthy Avocado Chicken Salad 150

Asian Edamame Salad, With Cilantro & Toasted Almonds 151

Crustless Spinach Bacon Quiche 152

Bacon Lettuce Tomato Spring Rolls 154

Shawarma Chicken Bowls - Basil-Lemon Vinaigrette 157

Thai Stuffed Avocados 159

Buffalo Chicken Lettuce Wraps 160

Big Fat Nori Wraps 162

Stir Fry with Keto Asian Cabbage 165

Soup with low carbohydrate stuffed peppers 167

Easy Keto Pad Thai 169

Cucumbers Caesar 171

SNACK RECIPES 172

Chicken Zucchini Poppers 172

Parmesan Garlic Zucchini Chips 174

Healthy Baked Broccoli Tots 174

Low Carb Cheese Crackers Recipe 176

Keto Big Mac Bites 179

Cauliflower Tots in Cheesy Baked 181

Chapter 1: What Is Carb Cycling And How Do You Get It?

Carb cycling is nothing but eating more carbohydrates for a specific number of days. These are called "High carb days" and promote muscle growth. Surplus days are "Low carb", which means that fewer carbohydrates have been consumed. This is intended to promote fat loss and minimize fat gain.

Is it possible to eat bread and still lose fat? Learn how you can curb your carbohydrate cravings to lose more fat.

Many people will repeat the mantra: Carbohydrates, can't live without them but can't live with it. Bread, pasta, potatoes, etc. are the first foods to be banned when weight loss is the goal. But, as we all know, a big bowl full of chips is just as good as eating pasta and potatoes. What would your reaction be if you were informed that more carbohydrates could actually increase fat loss

It is crucial that you understand that not all diets will work for you. However, once you realise that you are unable to eat certain foods, you can give up on any potential long-term weight loss. Don't worry, there are still ways you can shed those unwanted pounds.

If you understand the confusion around carbohydrates, you will soon be able to enjoy them and all their benefits instead of being afraid. You have now found the solution. This is due to a clever diet trick known as carbcycling. It allows all participants to get enough fuel, to fight the fat, but most importantly to enjoy their food.

It all boils down to the chain reaction

Carb cycling is about balancing between low and high carbohydrate diets. This is how carb cycling works. Your body will burn fat and keep you fueled.

Promoting lean muscles is crucial if you're looking to lose fat. However, low-calorie diets don't always support the body in its efforts to build it. Carb cycling is a great way to burn fat while building lean muscle. It has been shown that calorie and carbohydrate intake is essential to build lean muscle and improve health. Weight loss is not easy. However, consuming fewer calories and carbohydrates will force your body to use up its fat reserves. You can lose your strength and energy if you follow a low carb diet for too long. Carb cycling is a way to lose weight and still have the energy and strength of a high carb diet.

Food is the most important thing in your life.

We all know that carbohydrates are an important component of a healthy diet. It would be foolish to cut them out. It is vital to eat only the best food. This will only lead to poor health and weight gain.

High-carbohydrate food, including white pasta, white bread, sugary sweets, promote insulin production which can then lead to fat gain. It is the body's way of telling cells to store energy instead of using it. Insulin can then lead to an increase in fat stores.

It may sound like food substitutions with high-fat scratch foods will help you lose weight. But sugar-filled foods promote insulin production, so replacing these foods with low-fat ones will not work for your weight loss goals. You can also be at risk of developing diabetes or obesity from high-GI, processed foods.

People who have tried to follow a low-calorie diet, low-fat diet or low-carbohydrate diet to stay fit and healthy will know the unpleasant side effects. These include:

1) Poor concentration

2) Short temper

3) Mood swings

A carbohydrate cycling program can provide many benefits for their mental health, including the ability to quickly process information and improve their mental outlook. For brain function, glucose is vital. Research has shown that ketones are produced from fat and are used to fuel brain function. Ketosis is a state where you're eating low-carbohydrate diets to lose weight. You may find that mixing up your carbohydrate intake is a good idea for both your brain and your body.

Carb cycling is a great way to save money

There are some who recommend eating two days of low-carbohydrate meals and one high-carbohydrate day alternately. You can however switch between the two any other day. Keep in mind that your toughest workout days will have high carbohydrate days. So that your glycogen stores are replenished, you can eat the highest carbohydrate meal following your session. This should give you energy and refueling.

It doesn't really matter how low or high your carbohydrate diet is, getting enough protein is crucial. Your protein intake should be evenly distributed across all your meals. Protein is essential because it helps slow down blood sugar spikes caused by carbs. It also keeps you fuller longer and will aid in recovery from exercise. Protein sources include eggs, beef and chicken as well as oily fish such sardines or salmon. Also, you can include high-quality protein powders such whey protein isolates as well as brown rice.

These low carbohydrate days must be countered by eating plenty of healthy oils. Low-fat diets and restricting carb intake will result in feeling empty, hungry, and dissatisfied. You must keep your energy levels up, your stomach full, as well as your brain focused, if you intend to follow this plan. Good fats include linseeds (olive oil, avocado, coconut, oil, seeds, nuts and coconut oil). All of these products are high-in omega 3 and

6 fatty acids as well as vitamin E. These are all proven to be beneficial in weight loss.

Top tips to make carbohydrates work better for you

These top tips will help to explain how carbohydrates can be used to your advantage.

Change

It is possible to feel moody or have headaches after you switch to carb-cycling. Your body will adjust to using fats, proteins and carbohydrates for fuel. There's no danger. This is simply a metabolic adjustment.

Both odd and even

Try to maintain a balance of high carbohydrate and low carbohydrate day that is appropriate for your exercise program. This might mean that you may need to have moderate carbohydrate day. This formula will calculate how many grams of carbohydrates you should eat.

Low carb days: 0.6 grams x body weight, in pounds

High carb days: 1.4g x weight in pounds

Forward planning

It is a good idea to always have snacks on hand in case you run out of food options. You might consider taking a fibre supplement if it is difficult for you find healthy foods.

Cheat

Yes, that's right! You can keep your body guessing by having a cheat day, where you forget about your carb cycling plan for a week or more. As this will reduce the harm, cheat days should not be planned when you have an intense activity to complete.

Chapter 2: The Theory Behind Carbcycling

Understanding the theory behind weight loss is essential. You can explain carb cycling as follows. Your high-carbohydrate days refuel your muscles glycogen and flood your body's insulin which has an Anti-Catabolic effect. Anti-catabolic means that you release the amino acids into your bloodstream slowly as opposed to flooding. This will prevent the blood aminos levels from dropping below the required level.

You can allow your body to store glycogen as you provide fuel for the day. This will help to prevent weight loss.

People claim that magic happens for low carbohydrate days. Your insulin levels should be low to trick your body into burning fat more quickly.

Let's examine the science behind carbcycling. Is it possible to lose fat with a carbcycling diet? This is the obvious question. The answer is simple: yes.

No matter which weight loss plan you are on, weight loss will occur whether your body is in a calorific surplus daily, weekly or monthly.

It is important to remember that weight loss can be achieved if your body uses less energy than it needs.

The best thing about the carb cycle is their claim that there is no need to count calories and that you can eat whatever you want. Only one thing is needed to follow a set if rules. These rules are designed around eating lots of carbohydrate for high days, less for moderate days, and very little or no carbohydrate for low days. This type diet is very effective for maintenance. It can also be useful for weight loss.

A person must closely plan and monitor his macronutrient intake to keep body fat below 8 to 9 % for men and 18 - 19 % for ladies. This is crucial as they must be aware of how much protein and carbohydrate they are consuming each day.

This raises the question: is carb cycling better for weight management than traditional dieting?

Individuals who are enthusiastic about carb cycling will argue that it will dramatically accelerate fat loss when you eat less carbohydrate than traditional diets. However, science does not support these claims.

We can look at the University of Pennsylvania's study of 60 adults that followed the following diets.

Low-carbohydrate high-protein high-fat diet. 20g of carbohydrate was consumed per day. The amount was gradually increased to reach a desired weight.

OR

A conventional diet, where 60% of calories came from carbohydrates, 25% was from fat, and 15% from protein

The results showed that while the low-carbohydrate group gained more weight over the first 3 months, the overall difference over one year was not very significant.

It's not hard to see the difference after 3 months. This is especially true when you consider that by reducing carbs, you are decreasing your water retention as well as the amount of glycogen in the liver and muscles. This reduces total water retention. This alone will lead to a rapid decline in weight, but it has nothing whatsoever to do with burning calories.

Let's examine a Harvard University study about diet composition, weight loss and other topics. Researchers gave over 800 overweight adults the following diets.

1) 20% calories come from fat, 15% comes from protein, and 65% comes from carbohydrate

2) 40% from fat, 15% of protein and 45% for carbohydrate

3) 40% from fat, 25% of protein, and 35% from carbohydrate

After six months, participants to each diet lost an average amount of 6kg. They started to regain their weight after about a month and lost an average 4kg after two years. Researchers concluded that diets that contained fewer calories led to weight loss.

Arizona State University further studied the effects of high-carbohydrate and low-fat diets on weight loss. They found that they were equally effective over an 8-week period as low carbohydrate and high-protein diets.

One study that was especially pertinent was a comparison of a ketogenic and traditional diets to see which one had a metabolic advantage.

Twenty overweight adults were randomly assigned one of these options for the study.

Ketogenic diet: 60% of calories are from fat, 35% from proteins, and 5% from carbohydrates

OR

Traditional diet, which includes 30% calories of fat, 30% protein and 40% carbohydrates

After six weeks, the following results were achieved:

1) There was no significant difference between total weight loss and weight gain

2) Both diets scored higher in hunger ratings. There was no difference between them, indicating that the claims of carb cycling as decreasing hunger better than traditional eating habits are not true.

3) While both the low carbohydrate and high-carbohydrate diets were being followed, energy

expenditure increased. The low carbohydrate diet provided no metabolic boost.

4) Insulin sensitivity was raised in both diets but there was no discernible difference.

This is yet more evidence against the low carbohydrate movement. It shows that weight reduction in and of itself will improve insulin sensitivity regardless how diet is designed.

Although there is some debate as to whether carbcycling can lead to individuals losing fat and building muscle, the current answer is not conclusive. But it's not carb cycling that would make it possible. This would depend on how well you are training and your genetics.

If an individual was to have the following profile, it would indicate that they are out of shape and have lots of fat to shed. If they hadn't lifted weights before or had never concentrated on lifting heavy weights, you can expect a result in which they lose both fat as well as build muscle. This is due to the body responding well in the first place to a diet and exercise program.

An advanced weight lifter, however, who has reached their full genetic potential, will not gain muscle or lose fat unless he or she is taking steroids. This does not mean that steroids should be used. They should instead aim to preserve their muscle.

Carb cycling claims that it has a metabolic advantage. It is claimed that following a high-carbohydrate day can stimulate muscle growth and shock the metabolism. But, there is little scientific evidence supporting this claim.

Insulin can be used to preserve lean body mass, but will not promote muscle growth. Your metabolism can be accelerated by eating more, but not to the point that you can burn the extra calories and fat.

In reality, there are too many people looking for quick fixes and all kinds of nonsense to get to their goals. When the only way to reach them is to do some hard work and calculate.

Are you interested in carb cycling?

Carb cycling might be an option if your body doesn't cope well with carbohydrates.

Chapter 3: How Carb Cycling Works.

Carb cycling involves a low carbohydrate diet, which includes high carbohydrate periods. Most people believe that low carbohydrate consumption for long periods of the day is beneficial. A low-carb diet can lead to temporary weight loss and muscle gain. It is impossible to eat this way all the time as your body depends on carbohydrates for its daily functions.

At the opposite end of the spectrum are those who promote high-carbohydrate lifestyles. Although high-carbohydrate eating habits can help speed up your metabolism, it is not the best for weight loss. Carb cycling is the perfect solution. This in-between type of diet gives you both low and higher carbohydrate intakes, while allowing you to maintain the muscle you have and lose body fat. Other benefits include the fact that you can maintain your strength and endurance throughout your entire program.

How it works

Carb cycling provides the body the fuel it needs in order to increase metabolism and decrease calorie intake. Day rotations are made between high carb and low carb days. There are generally three types of days. It's important to remember that not all people can eat zero carb.

You can arrange your carb cycle in many different ways. If you want to do the three days cycled, you have several options. It is possible to choose to have four low-carb days and six high carb days for the week. However, this should be done evenly so there are no back to back high days. You can adjust your approach to meet your own goals. One way to achieve carb cycling is to eat more carbohydrate on training or exercise days and less carbohydrate on lower intensity training days. While the carb cycling plan usually requires you to eat at least 6 times per day for this, there are other options. Make sure you keep your daily intake consistent no matter what day it is.

Protein

A carb cycling diet is one that emphasizes protein.

Let's take a look at this example:

A 200 lb male should not eat less than 33 grams of protein per day if they are getting 1 g of proteins for each pound of body weight. For a person following a five-meal plan, 40 g should be consumed per meal. 28 g is recommended for a seven-meal plan.

Fats

It is important to ensure that your dietary fat stays consistent throughout your entire plan.

Carbohydrates

This type diet focuses on daily manipulations of carbohydrate consumption. You'll see this from the name carbcycling. The diet features three types of days, and each day is limited to the amount of carbohydrates available.

Low carb days

You must calculate the proportion of carbohydrates to fat and protein to get the best results. Low carb will result in a higher intake of protein. Women should multiply the current body weight of their partner by 1.2. Men should multiply this figure by 1.5. This number will indicate the total amount of protein that is required each day. It can then be multiplied with 4 to determine the total calories that will come from protein sources. Fats can also easily be calculated by multiplying the woman's weight by

0.58 and that of a man by 0.55. The total number multiplied by 9 will give you your fat-calorie consumption. It is possible to find carbohydrate calories by multiplying a woman's weight with 0.6 and a men's by 0.9. You can then add all three numbers together for your daily calorie consumption during this particular cycle.

Day of high carbohydrate

This is how high carb days are established. You use exactly the same method but increase your protein, carbohydrate intake and decrease your fats. To calculate the grams protein and carbohydrate, a woman needs to multiply her body weight by 1.44 and a male by 1.7. The fat grams can be calculated by multiplying the woman's body weight with 0.3 and the man's weight with 0.6. This gives you an indication of the number of nutrient dense calories that must be consumed each day.

No carb days

It is not the easiest day, but it is also the most mentally and physically demanding. It means that there are no carbohydrates. However, you will still get some carbs from greens. But not enough to negatively impact your results. The going won't be easy on no carb day, but it is possible to achieve great results if one can persevere. There are some people that can handle low carb days better than others. You'll be the one who decides whether or not to have carbs. This will depend on how you feel. Also, make sure you can function normally during the day. It's up to you to adjust your plan to meet your goals.

Chapter 4: Carb Cycling Facts And Fatloss

Carb cycling has become more popular and is growing in popularity. However, it is crucial that you understand all the details about carb cycling.

Many people who have looked at a wide range of information on fat loss diets have probably come across the carbohydrate cycle diet plan. This diet plan mixes high carb days with low carb days to aid in weight loss.

The side effects can include decreased exercise performance and increased hunger.

Some of these issues can be offset by increasing the carbohydrate day. Most people find this approach much more enjoyable. A few important facts are essential to remember before you start the carb cycling program. These are the following:

Heavy training should only be done on days with high carbohydrate intake

This is the key thing you should remember when designing your carbohydrate cycling program. You should do your hardest work on the carbohydrate-rich days. This is because your body needs these carbohydrate days. Consuming carbohydrates before you exercise will fuel your body to be able work harder, lift more weight and produce glycogen to aid recovery. Timing is key if you want all the carbohydrates to perform at their highest potential and not turn to body fat.

Water weight gain is to be expected

Another thing you should know is that your body will likely experience weight gain from higher carbohydrate diets. The body stores 4g of water for each gram of carbohydrate consumed. If you are eating 300g of carbohydrate, it will quickly add up.

Water weight gain will be more noticeable in the person who is leaner. This is normal, and it's not a cause for concern. However, you should notice a decrease in weight within a week or so of returning to a low-carbohydrate diet. People who have trouble with weight difference may not find carbohydrate cycling helpful. While the fluctuations in weight you will experience are something you can manage, they do not necessarily mean that it is something you should avoid.

Complex carbohydrates/carbohydrates high in glucose

Carb cycling is a great way to lose weight and you need to be mindful of the carbs. You need to avoid fructose because this carbohydrate behaves differently and doesn't offer the same benefits. High-carbohydrate diets may result in body fat gain if fructose is consumed frequently.

On high-carbohydrate days, reduce the fat

Your carb cycling diet should include reducing your overall dietary fat intake during high-carbohydrate meals. It's not unusual to increase your overall calories on a high-carbohydrate diet day. However, by decreasing your fat intake, you make more room for carbohydrates without going crazy with calories.

It is best to limit your intake of carbohydrate on your low carbohydrate diet to between 300-600 calories. If you plan to have a low-calorie, very low carb day, this will help to reduce the weight loss.

To lose fat, keep your calorie target level.

The equivalent of 15,400 calories per workweek is 2200 calories per day. To lose 1 Pound, you must make a 3,500 calorie calorie deficit each week. You can do this by simply increasing your food intake to 11,900 Calories. A standard diet will allow you to eat the same calorie intake on every day. That would translate into 1700 calories per daily (2200-500 = 1700).

Carbohydrate cycling is a process where you need high-carbohydrate diet days to have more calories. Therefore, it is important to know the mass. The remaining 4,700 calories for these three days is 7,200, or roughly 1,200 calories per day.

This is because low carbohydrate diets have less calories. However, you may find that this doesn't seem to be a problem if you come off a high-carbohydrate diet. If you don't want to bring your low-calorie day down, adjust the intake for high carb days so that you get more calories for the low-carb days.

Balance at the end is all about finding the right balance.

Now that you know all the details, you can start carbohydrate-cycling. This is a great way to help maintain performance and avoid weight loss plateaus. To ensure you adhere to the set intakes, you will need to take more time.

Chapter 5: Advanced Fat Loss, And Why Carb Cycling Works

Although it is obvious that carb cycling works, the question remains: why? Carb cycling can help you lose body fat quickly and without affecting your muscle mass. There are many drawbacks to low-carb diets. Carb cycling can be a difficult diet strategy. It requires commitment and is not suitable for anyone looking to lose a few weight quickly. Carb cycling is appropriate for:

1) You are above the age 18

2) You are in good health

3) You have strong will power and are not tempted to cheat

If you answered no to any one of the above, basic calorie count for healthy eating and your daily exercise will be sufficient. It is important that you remember that losing fat without removing muscles is more difficult than getting leaner. However, carb cycling can help.

Carb cycling can be a difficult fitness method. It requires more than hard work and dedication. But it is the only way that you can burn body fat and maintain muscle. Once you have created your customized meal plan and determined what you need to do to begin your own carb-cycling strategy, you will quickly see why this method is so hard for motivated people. You cannot help but count, weigh, and track the nutritional value of every food item you consume.

There are many factors that make carb cycling successful. Although it is possible that the cycling of carbs will not help you that much it is possible, the fact is that this program is scientifically supported and can be used to lose fat fast while losing very little muscle.

Tom Venuto (creator and expert of the carbcycling diet) and Will Brink ("expert") have written remarkable books about how to lose fat and provide far more information than you can imagine on how to carb cycle fat loss.

Many people wonder how long they should keep on the carb-cycling diet. The short answer is until they have achieved their goal. Carb cycling is for those who want to lose weight and get back to healthy eating. It's personal preference. Many carbcyclists have made it their way of life.

Why it works

Cycling carbs is more a hormonal way of eating than a calorific one. Numerous hormones, which influence the way your body is formed, are affected by your carbohydrate intake.

Insulin

Insulin is both a fat-storing and muscle building hormone. In order to aid the metabolism, insulin is released into bloodstream.

When it comes to insulin and carb consumption, the main point to remember is to eat to your satiety level and not to overeat. Insulin release depends on how much carbs you eat. Carb cycling, however, manipulates insulin to limit fat storage while making the most muscle synthesis.

Leptin

Leptin is most commonly produced by fat cells. Leptin can be released when you consume high amounts of carbohydrate and high calories. Leptin is not affected by insulin. Leptin slowly increases as a result of increased carbohydrate consumption. Leptin goes to the hypothalamus and signals that you're full. Secondary hormones, such as leptin, also feed into the hypothalamus.

Leptin sends the signal to your body to speed up metabolism.

Leptin levels can remain high in people who consume a high carbohydrate and high calorie diet. This can lead the hypothalamus not to be able hear leptin, which can result in leptin resistance. If this happens, we don't feel satisfied and it can lead to weight gain. The body will respond by sending very low levels, or even zero, of leptin when it is eating a low-calorie, low carbohydrate diet. Carb cycling can lead to leptin causing a rapid increase in hunger and slowing down the metabolism. High-carbohydrate days are necessary to help the body reset.

Serotonin

Serotonin is sometimes called the "sanityhormone" and it is a feeling-good brain chemical that boosts mood. Doctors and other health professionals use it often to treat depression. Because carbohydrates increase serotonin production, eating carbohydrates can boost mood.

Low serotonin results from a low carbohydrate lifestyle and can cause increased food cravings, such as for sugar or chocolate. Low serotonin is a major reason diets often fail. Carb cycling restores and regulates your serotonin level. It makes it less difficult to have cravings. Individuals who carb cycle find it easier to stick with than other diets, as their serotonin levels don't drop completely.

Cortisol

Cortisol is an inverted hormonal which means it can break down molecules so they can be used for fuel. Cortisol's ability to be both beneficial and destructive can be due to its inability to distinguish between muscle and fat-burning for fuel. Multiple studies have demonstrated that eating protein can help maintain muscle in catabolic states.

Consuming carbohydrates can reduce cortisol, which is why bodybuilders prefer to eat carbs as well as protein within the first hour of waking up. Excess cortisol is prevented by following a carb cycle program. This is because high carb days can help reset the hormone at the time when it starts producing excessive amounts.

Chapter 6: Breaking Through The Diet Plateau

Many people decide to drop body fat and get a phenomenal body.

Initial fat loss is far and away the easiest.

The best way to cut fat is initially simple. While there are many diets out there, carb cycling is proven to be effective. It is based on high quality food choices and maintaining a relative calorie surplus to start and maintain fat loss. Your personal activity level and metabolic factors will influence your unique carb cycling plan. It is up to you then to choose the best method for you.

Stop analysing if you have excess body fat. Start moving! Don't complicate or be confused by things. Start moving right away!

The linear diet problem

But reaching your final destination can be a lot more complicated. Planning your meals will require you to be more organized. As you will have less fat, you'll be able to make more mistakes. In fact, this is the point where you're at greatest risk of losing muscle mass or sabotaging metabolic function by using poor dieting.

The linear method of diet where you reduce calories every day until you reach your goal is not very effective. It can, however, lead to enormous weight gains as your diet returns more to normal.

The human body is an adaptive organism that can adapt to any calorific deficiency. In the end, however, the more you diet, the more likely it will become difficult to achieve results and eventually you will hit a plateau. This is because of a hormone called Leptin, which slows down when there is calorific restriction. Lower levels of leptin may lead to more hunger cravings. It will also slow down the metabolism rate and decrease energy expenditure. This is why it is not a good combination to lose fat and maintain it. Leptin is a master controlling hormone. It can cause changes in other hormones, so if you are in a calorie deficit, there may be drastic drops in your testosterone and growth hormones.

The cycling solution

The opposite effect of cutting calories is when you overfeed your body. Overeating for two days can result in a slowing of the metabolism that is commonly seen in dieting. This can help to restore pre-diet levels of leptin hormone, testosterone and growth hormone.

You can see why many get confused when trying to find a way to reduce fat, maintain muscle and avoid falling into the hormonal and metabolic traps of extreme dieting. Use carb cycling in conjunction with calorie control. What you really need are some strategies to re-sensitize and push through that plateau to burn stubborn fat. Get rid of that extra layer of fat that seemed to be holding on for dear. There are many effective dieting strategies. Here are some to think about:

The 5/2

One plan suggests that those with body weight to lose be in calorie deficiency for 5 days a semaine. This diet should contain between 10 and 12 calories for each pound of weight. This is suitable for both training or rest days.

You should consume more calories the second day, ideally around 20 calories per kg. These two days are where you should be doing your most intense training. Leptin levels rise when your carbs increase. It is better to get your carbohydrates from carbohydrates than protein or fat. In other words, the carbs rise while the protein and fat levels remain the same.

The 3/4

If you are looking to lose weight but improve the quality of your life, it is important to cycle your days so that the low-calorie days can burn fat while the high-calorie days support muscle recovery and growth.

The goal is to work towards your maintenance caloric level. For an average person, this would be around 15 calories per kilogram. If you choose to take a day off and are not doing any activity, then you should consume calories that are more geared towards fat loss. These calories would need approximately 10 - 12 calories for each pound of body weight. To build muscle mass, the calories for active workouts must be increased to 18 calories per pound. The calories should be accompanied by more carbohydrates.

How low can you go with carbs?

When you're engaged in intense exercise, it is best to continue eating starchy carbohydrates even when you're at rest. For intense exercise, carbs are vital for supporting your body's needs.

Studies have shown that glycogen recovery takes place after exercise for longer periods of time. According to me, glycogen restoration can take place for more than three hours after a workout.

There are several types of calorie cycling. All the above plans qualify as carb biking because they require the fat, protein and calorie intake to be constants and the increase to come from carbs.

However, there are those who recommend greater fluctuations in carbohydrates and the accompanying increase or decrease in dietary cholesterol to compensate. Based on research and studies, the following sums up true carb cycling.

1. Rest/low-calorie days: Eat a low-carbohydrate diet, with the carbs coming mainly from vegetables and whole fruit. You should avoid starches, and the remainder of your daily calorie requirement should be fulfilled by dietary fat.

2. You can eat low fat/high carbohydrate combinations on your higher-calorie days. You should get your fat from lean proteins and not add more fats. Your remaining calorie

requirements   should   be   fulfilled   by
carbohydrates.

Finally

You can see that diets vary from person to person and there is no single universal way. The strategies listed here are just a starting point. You will need to try many different ones before you finally find what works for your needs.

Chapter 7: Carb Cycling To Help You Lose Weight

A lot of questions will be raised about carb cycling for weight loss.

1) Is carbocycling different from other weight loss techniques?

2) Can you really expect carb cycling to help you lose weight?

3) What benefits does carb cycling offer?

You need to understand that carb cycling will not help you lose weight faster than any other type of diet. There are many options for diets, and most will yield results if they are followed consistently.

Here lies the problem: your inability to stick to the diet. Many diets are restrictive in your food choices, or so bad that you feel miserable you don't want to eat.

To answer the questions above:

1) Carb Cycling is different in that it does not restrict any macronutrient, and can be incorporated into a lifestyle modification because there is no expiry.

2) You shouldn't set any unrealistic goals to lose weight.

3) Carbocycling is a great way to lose weight and satisfy your mind.

Why it works

To understand why carb cycling works, it is necessary to first understand why some diets fail. We will examine the main reasons and explain how carb cycling can help overcome those potential failures.

Not eating enough

The majority of diets will cause a calorie shortage, which is then maintained for the duration. Carb cycling is an exception because it allows you to combine low-calorie days with high-calorie ones. This helps to reset your metabolism and prevent starvation mechanisms becoming too dominant, which can lead to failure.

You're not changing your lifestyle, you're just dieting

The common thread in all diets is that they end. You feel the same as when you began them. This is not the case with carb cycling. Instead of being a diet, you can incorporate it into your lifestyle.

Manufactured nutrients are lacking

If you eat foods that contain the three most important macronutrients, you have the best chance of getting all of your essential vitamins and mineral requirements to build muscle mass and reduce fat.

Foods made from diet are bland and tasteless

Dieting can lead to bad tasting food. This is because most people believe they need restrict the intake of certain foods.

Carb cycling is not only good for carbs but also encourages high carbohydrate days. Let's be real, most people love carbs.

Slow weight loss

It is best to not jump on the scales while carb cycling. To track your progress, you need to get into the habit for measuring or wearing tight clothes. You should do this because carbs can cause extreme weight swings. You can lose weight if you eat too many carbohydrates. This happens because water attaches itself to the sugar molecules of the carbohydrates. It is possible to lose weight quickly if you control your calorie intake.

You long for control

Most likely, you've tried a no-carb diet. However, while some may find this to be the ideal approach, most people found that they were more hungry and more difficult forgiving. You can reduce your appetite suppression and satiety hormones by following a high carbohydrate diet.

Carb cycling meal planning

Are you now familiar with the concept of carbcycling? Do you want to know how to get started?

The basic idea behind this is to cycle your carbohydrate intake, so that you have both high and low days. There are many options for how you can cycle carbs. It is important to tailor your diet to your needs.

Here are some examples.

- Low low, low high, high low, low high, low high, and low high - repeat

- Low and high, high, lower, high, repeat

- Low low high low low high, low high, high high low, hi, low high, low high, low again

It is so easy! But which one is best? Consider the following guidelines when planning your individual plan.

1) It is important to have high carbohydrate days in conjunction with high-intensity workout days

2) Plan low-carbohydrate days on cardio or rest day.

These are just a few of the many benefits you get from taking these points into account.

There is a good chance you are curious as to what your daily routine and meals look like. It is recommended to have a consistent protein intake, regardless of day. You can increase your carbohydrate intake on low-carb days while decreasing your high-carb days. The following are some general guidelines that you could choose to use:

- In general, eat between 0.8 gram and 1 gram protein per pound of body weight

- You should consume 50/50 calories from fat and protein on low carb days. However, you don't need to eat any carbs.

You should consume between 400 and 600 grams of carbs on high-carb days. The body will reset its metabolism and hunger hormones by increasing calories to levels higher than the maintenance level. Keep fat down on these days because your insulin levels will go up and insulin is a storage hormone.

It is important that you experiment with the amount you can consume of high carbohydrate foods. Some people only have one high carbohydrate day per week while others choose to eat medium or low carbs the rest of the time. If you monitor your fat loss carefully, you can adjust things to fit your needs. Carb cycling is not a specific diet. However, once you master it the fat-loss potential can be incredible.

Chapter 8: Frequently Asked Questions

Every nutrition guide printed has included some form of carb cycling. Many of the top-respected sports coaches recommend carb cycling. Fitness models, athletes, and bodybuilders also use carb cycling to attain the most amazing bodies.

Although it is very popular in the fitness industry, carb cycling seems to be mysterious. People mistakenly assume that carb cycling is some complicated method. If done correctly, carb cycling is a great way to lose weight and enjoy carbs.

There are many diets that prohibit all carbohydrates. However, it is important for you to understand how carbohydrates affect your body. This is just one question that people often ask when considering carb cycling. Therefore, we have answered the following frequently-asked questions to ensure you have a solid understanding before you begin a carb cycle.

Qu 1 : How do carbohydrates impact the body?

Ans. When carbohydrates are consumed, they're broken down into sugars (more commonly called glucose) which then enter your blood stream.

The hormone insulin is then released in order to flush out the toxic glucose from our bloodstream. Eating simple refined sources like fruits, chocolates and fizzy drinks can lead to large insulin spikes. Conversely, a more complex source such vegetables and some grains will cause a smaller insulin spike.

Over the years, insulin has been responsible for most of obesity's problems. This belief states that insulin tells the body how to eliminate glucose from the bloodstream and to store it as a fat. However, it must be acknowledged that this isn't technically correct. Instead of telling the body to burn the glucose stored in the cells, insulin actually tells them to do so.

Carbohydrates, which provide energy instantaneously for all the cells in your body, are vital. Without carbohydrates, it's likely that your metabolism won't slow down and stress hormones will rise. Muscle building hormones will also plummet, making fatloss impossible.

If someone is very sedentary and works in an office, they will be most likely to be able to consume low carbohydrate food as their energy requirements are very low. For anyone who is active regularly, walks a lot, and likes to eat out often, carb cycling is the best option.

Qu 2 Why does carbocycling work?

Ans. Any diet that is effective will include elements of carb cycling. This is important because it simply involves changing the daily intake of carbohydrate in a structured manner.

You can cycle carbs in many ways. However, for simplicity's sake, you eat more carbs on one occasion and less the next. When you eat less carbs, fat burning is increased. Conversely, when you eat more carbs, you provide your body with the fuel it needs to function at its best. Carb cycling offers the best of both, and it is very easy to do.

Carb cycling can also mean that you are cycling calories. To lose weight, you need to have a calorie surplus. Carb cycling makes it simple to create this deficit.

As the body loses weight, it becomes more difficult for the body to burn fat. At this point, the body can go into starvation mode. This process is scientifically called adaptive thermo genesis. It's very real. By telling the body that it isn't starving, carb cycling can help to offset adaptive thermogenesis. This is how carb biking has helped so many people become lean.

Another factor that makes carbcycling work is that technically, you only have to eat certain days of each week.

Qu 3 - Should you eat Bread?

Ans. The answer will depend on whether or not you have a high carb day.

Qu 4 - What's a typical week for carb cycling?

Ans. This is a typical week for carb cycling.

Monday Full body exercise High Carb

Tuesday Rest Day Low Carb

Wednesday Full body work out High Carb

Thursday Rest Day Low Carb

Friday Full body work out High Carb

Saturday Rest day low carb

Sunday Rest Day Low Carb

Qu 5 - Can I still eat at restaurants?

Answer: If you're going out for dinner, plan your week so that you exercise on the day. This will reduce any chance of losing weight.

Qu 6 - What are good carbs, and what are bad carbs.

The following table shows you a summary of foods that can be classified as good or poor carbs.

Good Carbs and Poor Carbs

Sweet/white potatoes Pizza

Brown Rice Cakes

Quinoa Muffins

Wholegrain bread

Oatmeal Cereal

Whole-wheat Pastries

The better your body will function if you stick to good carbs.

Qu 7: What should I do if my low carb diet makes me hungry?

Ans. Because starchy carbs have lots of calories, they can fill you up quickly. This could make it difficult to feel full on low-carb days. It's much easier to succumb if you're hungry. You need to learn how to deal with this situation. Do not eat frozen pizzas. Instead, eat more vegetables.

Qu 8 - How many carbs should you have with every meal?

Ans. One of the best aspects about carb cycling, is its simplicity. There's no need to make it more complicated by counting how many carbs you consume. Be mindful:

High carb days: Choose fruit and starchy carbs as a complement to the protein, vegetable and fats

Low carb days: You can eat starchy carbs but not any fruit. Keep eating protein, vegetables and fats.

Do not complicate your meals. It's okay to eat more of the same every day.

Qu 9 Can I do high-carb day if I am only doing cardio?

Ans. High-carb days are best for days where you lift weights and do a bodyweight training. Your muscles will need to wait for the glucose to be available after a hard working out.

If you are trying to lose weight, it is best to stick with a conventional diet. It is important to include resistance training as part of your exercise routine in order to get the most out of high carb days.

Chapter 9: Get Started!

You've made the decision to eat healthy. A no carb diet won't help you. No matter what your ambitions, carb cycling could be the right choice for you.

Your metabolism will be kept efficient burning healthy carbohydrates by eating on specific days. In the meantime, you can fill up with protein and other vegetables on the days in between. This will help keep your insulin low enough so that you can lose fat without gaining muscle.

Now that you're curious, let us help you put together a carb cycle menu.

What's your recipe?

The most popular carb cycling plan will have you alternate between high- and low-carb cycling six days a weeks. Your seventh day can be reserved for treats or cheats, if necessary. You might want to vary the way you do things. If you're trying to lose weight, then you can have five low carb days while having high carbs on two of them. For those who are looking to gain muscle and weight, they might opt for 4-5 high carb days with the rest being low carb.

You should not have your high carb days all at once; they should be spread evenly through the week.

Whatever your plan, be sure to keep an eye on your progress and adjust your schedule if necessary to get the best results.

Consider your fuel

Many people fall for the false belief that they can eat meat on low carb days while eating pasta the rest. Research by the Academy of Nutrition and Dieticians shows that complex carbohydrates, such as whole grains and legumes, are the best way to get the most out of high carb days. They will keep you awake throughout the game and help you lose weight. You should aim to get your low-carb days' protein from lean chickens, fishes, beef, tofu, eggs, and then add non-starchy vegetables.

Take a snack to help you keep track of your goals

A majority of carb cycling followers and trainers recommend that you have a treat/cheat days where you can eat what you want. However, you must ensure it is not causing any setbacks.

It is best to avoid the weekly reward day if carb cycling is something you wish to make a habit of. You might get so used to thinking you can just eat whatever you like, and that you end up with a huge amount of calories that it will be difficult to continue the changes you have made.

It doesn't mean to be discouraged.

Meal plan

A meal plan/daily schedule is a great way to ensure you are stocked up with healthy proteins, grains, and produce. Although this is going to vary between people, women will need around 1,200 calories and men approximately 1,500 calories on low carb day. This can be slightly higher on high carb day. Many believe that the best way to calculate each macronutrient's portion is to work out how many grams are per pound of your bodyweight. These can be done using the following formulas.

Days of high carbohydrate

Men:

2 - 3g carbs for every kilo of your body weight

- 1 to 1.25 grams of protein x body weight

- Reduce as much fat as you can

Women:

Approximately 1 gram of carbs x your bodyweight

- 0.75 grams protein x your bodyweight

- Reduce as much fat as you can

Days with low carbohydrate

Men:

0.5 to 1.5 grams of carbs per kilogram body weight

1.25 - 1.5g protein x your bodyweight

- 0.15 to 0.35grams of fat x body weight

Women:

- 0.2 – 0.5 grams carb x your weight

About 1 gram of Protein x your Body Weight

- 0.1% - 0.2% of fat x your bodyweight

It is important to eat breakfast promptly after you wake up. You can then spread the calories out over the other meals.

Meal plan with high and low carbohydrate

Day of low carbohydrate:

7 a.m. 2 x scrambled Eggs with 1/2 Bell Pepper (red)

10 a.m.-protein shake with handfuls berries

1 p.m.-3.0 oz. Grilled chicken with asparagus

4 p.m. 1/3 cup oatmeal with handful (10) almonds

7 p.m.- 3 oz Steak with 2 cups of Broccoli and Cauliflower Steamed

A typical high-carb day

7 a.m.-1/2 cup oatmeal with walnuts and berries

10 a.m.- Apple with 2 Tbsp almond or peanut butter

1 p.m. 1/2 turkey sandwich on whole-wheat bread

4 p.m.-3 cup 3 bean salad, 1 cup quinoa

7 p.m.-3 oz grilled chicken, 1 cup whole wheat pasta, and pesto

Remember that you can still enjoy your favorite foods, but in moderation. The goal is to slowly change how you eat so that you include healthy foods. This will help you stick to your plan and ensure that you have long-term success.

Now that you know the basics of how to get healthier and leaner, you can take the first step towards becoming a better you.

Chapter 10: A 4 Week Carb Cycling Meal Plan

This chapter offers a variety of recipes and ideas to help you build your own custom plan. Your weekly schedule can be adapted to make your menu more flexible. You can also create a temporary calorie surplus to help you gain strength and lean mass.

These examples should not be taken as a guide. You will need additional information or to alter them to suit your specific needs.

A sample week of carb cycling

Day 1

Day 2: Low carb

Day 3 with low carbs

Day 4: High Carb Day

Low Carb Day 5

Day 6: Low Carb

High Carb Day 7

Low carb

Smaller portion of starchy foods and/or whole grain after work.

No workout drink required No workout drink required Work out drink No workout drink required No workout drink required Work out drink No workout drink required

No fruit No fruit 2 - 3 pieces of fruit No fruit No fruit 2 - 3 pieces of fruit No fruit

You should fill the rest the day full of lean protein and green vegetables.

You could also look at your week in the following way:

Monday Meal

Tuesday with high carbohydrate

Wednesdays low in carb

Medium carb Thursday

Friday with low carb

Saturdays low in carb

Sunday with high carbohydrate

Low carb

Breakfast 50g oats and 200ml skimmed Milk, Raspberry and Honey Ham omelette, Spinach and Goats Cheese omelette With Walnuts Scrambled eggs, lean bacon, and mushrooms Mushroom Omelette and handful Of Nuts 50g oats and 200ml Skimmed Milk, Raspberries and Honey Smoked Haddock fillet served with asparagus and 2 poached eggs

Snacks after workout, protein shake Carrot sticks, almond butter, and Cucumber, and carrot batons. Post-workout shake Cucumbers, carrot, and pepper batons.

Lunch 100g quinoa served with salmon fillet and half an avocado. Lamb steak with 1 sweet potato. Tuna and egg salad 100g. Quinoa with 2 eggs, chicken breast, and quinoa. Also, sliced lamb on skewers.

Snack Small saucepan of hummus and carrot, cucumber, celery sticks 2x boiled eggs Small saucepan of hummus and carrot, cube, and celerysticks Ham Salad Small Pot of hummus and carrot, with cucumber, celery sticks and celerysticks Baked sweet potatoes with sweetcorn and tuna Ham and avocado salad

Dinner Ginger chicken stir fry Steak served with roasted vegetables and cod fillet. Tuna steak with broccoli and cauliflower. Pork chops with various vegetables. Chili con carne, with rice and green veggies. Beetroots, spinach, and goat's cheese salad.

Snack Greek Greekyoghurt, cinnamon and nuts Greek Greekyoghurt Greekyoghurtwith cinnamonand walnuts Greek Greekyoghurtwith cinnamonand walnuts Greek Greekyoghurtwith cinnamonand walnuts Greek Greekyoghurtwith cinnamonand walnuts. Small bowl of porridge with Greek Greekyoghurt and cinnamon Greekyoghurtwith cinnamonand walnuts

A weekly plan another option that you might be interested in following could be the one below:

Alternatives to high-protein, low-carb diets

Meal Protein Carbs Fibrous Vegetables Fat

Breakfast 2 egg whites and one whole egg with 3oz ground Turkey, beef, or chopped Ham to create an omelette 1/2 Grapefruit or 1/3 cup oatmeal Omelette style vegetables like onion and green peppers. Fat is found in the meat and egg yolk

Mid-morning 2 scoops of low-carb protein powder to make a shake 2 Tbsps peanut butter

Lunch 5 oz chicken/turkey/6 oz fish, grilled 1 cup green vegetable 1 - 2 Tsp flaxseed Oil plus the fat from the meat

Mid Afternoon 6oz can tuna and chicken or low carb Protein Bar Celery or Carrots

Supper: 5oz steak, chicken/turkey, or fish; 2 cups spinach leaves. 1 tbsp olive or vinegar dressing.

An alternative option to the above meal plan is to keep the low carb diet in place every day, and then alternate days, such as Wednesday or Saturday, when you replace the last supper meal with one the following high carbohydrate meals:

Meal Protein Carbs Fibrous Vegetables Fat

High Carb: 1 1/2 oz sweet potato, 1/3 cup of oatmeal, small banana, 1 cup of vegetables (spinach, green beans, broccoli, etc.) 1 tsp butter, flax seed or oil

High Carb 1/2 cup whole grain pasta or 1/2 Cup brown rice with 2 tablespoons with 1 cup vegetable such as spinach green beans, asparagus, and broccoli 1 teaspoon butter or flax oil

Meal Protein Carbs Fibrous Vegetables Fat

High Carb2 cont 2 tbsp Marinara Sauce, 4 strawberries or raspberries

High Carb 3 Low fat chili, with or without meat

Another option is to follow the Low Carb Plan and then, over time, modify your meals to include more complex carbs throughout each day.

Meal Protein Carbs Fibrous Vegetables Fat

Breakfast 2 x eggwhites, 1 whole eggs and 6 oz skimmed dairy 1/3 cup oatmeal.

Mid Morning 1/2 cup lowfat yoghurt or 8oz milk. Then add 1 scoop of protein powder to the milk.

Lunch 4oz turkey/ turkey breast or 5oz fish 4oz sweetness potato 1 cup green vegetable 1 tsp flaxseed oil plus any fats in the meat

Mid-afternoon 4oz cans tuna, chicken or half a cup pinto beans. 1 slice whole grain bread. 1 medium Apple. 1 tsp flaxseed Oil

Supper 4oz chicken and turkey, fish or lean meat 4oz sweet potato or 1/2 c brown rice 1 c green vegetables Fat within the meat

Important points to remember about carb cycling

Your activity and calorie needs should be considered when determining your approach.

- Decide on your preferred high or low carb day in advance. Keep to this

- Don't stop making decisions based upon your results

High Carb Days - For the best results in body composition, do some exercise

- Plan your high-carb days with this in mind: The body can tolerate carbs well when you are active in the morning, or first thing in your day.

You can get an extra boost by adding this to your shopping cart

Carb cycling is a good way to manage leptin or ghrelin. These hormones regulate appetite and body composition.

Carb cycling maximizes glycogen stores and makes it easier to work out during low calorie periods. You will get less fiber if your carbohydrate intake is lower. In this instance, it is crucial to eat a lot of high fiber foods and drink enough water to avoid constipation.

The final words

1) Only use carbcycling if you are absolutely certain that it's the right eating plan.

2) Decide your own strategy. This will be determined by how you feel about low carb days. How much muscle you have. Your physique. Also, this will determine if this is a lifestyle change and how long you can sustain carb cycling.

3. Once you have settled on your strategy, you can start to calculate your calorie intake

4) You should establish your calories and determine your protein intake. This should not change from your fat goal.

5) Set your carbohydrate intake goals on high and low carb day

6) Last, you should divide all the other essential nutrients into the appropriate meal plan

61

7) You can now decide which days are high carb and get ready to go

8) Feel great, start, and sustain!

Chapter 11: The Origin Of Carb Cycling & The Low Carb Diet

Low-carb diets strictly limit your intake of carbs. These diets can be used to treat obesity. Low-carb diets essentially restrict the consumption of high-carbohydrate foods and allow for foods rich in protein and fat. But, some foods can be allowed.

Low Carb Diets Increasing in Popularity

William Banting, from London, England, wrote and published the 1863 book, Letter on Corpulence. It is the book that launched the low-carb revolution. He explained how low carb diets helped him lose weight.

To promote ketosis, the body decreases insulin production by reducing the nutritive carbohydrates. Ketosis is a state in which the body uses the fat stored as energy to lose weight faster.

The Dilemma: The Problems with Low Carb Diets in Relation to Their Benefits

While low-carb diets have proven to be effective in weight loss, as well as for treating other diseases, such diabetes, high blood pressure, and heart disease, there have been controversies and criticisms throughout the years.

Because of their ability to lose weight in two weeks or less, strict low-carb diets became very popular. Medical research has shown that this type diet can increase your risk of developing cardiovascular disease. People who have tried this diet reported that they gained weight much quicker after the reintroduction carbs. You can get the benefits of fast fat loss and still have the energy for intense training to build muscle.

Below are additional issues that can be associated with low carb diets.

- Dehydration is a short-term problem that dieters will have to deal with when the program starts early. The loss of water in the body accounts for most of the weight that you will lose during your low-carb diet.

- You may feel fatigue or weakness after a few weeks of low carb dieting. This is because the body still needs to adjust to the reduced intake of carbs. Low-carb diets shouldn't be mixed with any exercise programs. The good news is that, once the body has adjusted, it will not be affected by the diet.

- Low-carb diets are causing concerns about the intake of vegetables and fruits high in carbohydrates. Nutritionists claim that restricting your intake of fruits, vegetables, and other nutrients not only reduces the supply but also lowers your ability to absorb vitamins and mineral. While some fruits and vegetables have low carbohydrate content are allowed to be eaten, it is still a matter of debate whether low-carb diets are safe for the health of dieters.

Many people believe that low-carb diets are dangerous because they require multi-vitamins or supplements. Multi-vitamins, supplements, and multivitamins can be helpful in helping the body adapt to sudden drops in carbohydrate supplies.

Low-carb diets can work, there's no doubt about that. For some, however, this type of diet may prove too difficult and restrictive to be maintained. For those who exercise or do strength training, low-carb eating is not recommended.

Carb Cycling: A Better Alternative

Carb cycling was born out of these criticisms and limitations. The Carb Cycling movement is controversial. Franco Carlotto may be the one to credit for the Carb Cycle, which is a method of eating carbs in a healthy way. Carlotto won six Mr. World Fitness Titles. This has enabled thousands of people to be fit.

Some claim that carb cycling was first covered in The Ketogenic Diet by Lyle Macdonald. This sports nutrition enthusiast is now a highly respected fitness professional. The concept of ketogenic diets was not new, although Macdonald wrote the book.

Carbcycling is a low carb diet that alternates between high and low carbohydrate intake. This diet is intended to lose weight effectively while maintaining your energy level to exercise and do intense workouts. Carb cycling works in the same way as the regular low-carb lifestyle. It limits how much carbohydrate you consume depending on where you are at the moment. This diet encourages your body to remain in ketosis. Your body then consumes all of its remaining calories through foods high in fats and protein.

The following chapter will discuss the principles of carbcycling: how it works to eliminate excess fats, and how you can make use of it to support your bodybuilding routine.

Chapter 12: The Fundamental Principles Of Carb Cycling

Although the idea of carb cycling was first introduced to the public, it has been used by bodybuilders for years. While bodybuilders bulk up, they would eat lots of carbs and then use the carb cycling method to lose the excess fats. The bodybuilders found it to be a very effective technique, so personal trainers began testing it on non-bodybuilders. The results were amazing.

Effectiveness - Just the Right Carb Amounts

The carb cycling diet proved effective and was gradually introduced to more fitness lovers, especially to those who regularly go to the gym. You should eat enough carbohydrates to fuel you for exercise and training while still losing fats and making progress towards your weight loss goals.

Carb Cycling in Two Phases

There are two types of carb cycling days, high-carb day and low-carb. The body receives more carbs during the high-carb days. This makes it more ready to exercise and train. The body is also replenished with glycogen, which helps stimulate the muscles. This allows it to perform more challenging activities throughout the day. The body can be tricked into burning bodyfats for energy during low-carb diet days.

The Carb Cycling Diet is a fat-burning and muscle building diet.

In order to provide enough energy for your daily activities, the body will enter ketosis when it has been starved of carbohydrate supplies during low-carb weeks. The body will burn extra fats to produce energy and help you lose weight. In terms of muscle building, low-carb diets can trim excess fat and prepare the body for high-carb diets.

Your body will replenish nutrients lost during low carb days as the high-carb weeks approach. Your muscles will be ready for as many carbs and as little as possible during this period. Without having to eat too much food or supplement, your muscles will grow by being able to absorb carbohydrates.

The carb refills that are given once or twice per week address issues such as fatigue, weakness (dehydration), hunger pangs, fatigue, and fatigue. The dieter may consume more carbohydrates during high-carb weeks than they would on a low- or normal-carb day. The main purpose of carb refill days is to:

1. To replenish glycogen stores (in muscle and liver), that have been reduced by intense activities or exercise sessions.

2. To normalize thyroid activity and other hormones the body was deprived of during low carb days.

3. To give you a break from your daily routine.

Refilling glycogen stores in the body can allow dieters to increase their endurance and build muscle, something that would not be possible on a strictly low carb diet. But, high-carb days are risky if not closely monitored. The carb refill can lead to a person gaining more weight if they consume more carbohydrates than needed to replenish their glycogen stores. You need to watch the time and frequency of carb replenishment days. It is also important to ensure proper nutrition allocation to keep your body balanced.

The following chapter will explain how to make your own carb-cycling pattern. It will also help you create the best plan to achieve your goals.

Chapter 13: Carbohydrate Patterning

Carb cycling has many unique features. This diet can be adjusted to meet any workout regimen and any fitness goals. There are many different carb cycling patterns a dieter could choose from. Below are some examples of simple patterns that would be suitable for someone who lives an active, healthy lifestyle.

The Classic Cycle

The carb-cycling model will allow a person to have alternating high and low carbohydrate days, with the seventh day as a reward. Example: A dieter may start his diet program Monday and make it a low-carb day. The next day, Tuesday should be high-carb and Wednesday should also be low-carb. He will continue this process until Sunday, which is the reward.

For low-carb diets, 1500cal is recommended for men and 1200cal per woman. However, high-carb days have a suggested calorie intake of 2000cal for men and 1500cal for ladies. Reward days allow dieters to eat as much as they like, as long as their calorie intake does no exceed 3000cal or 2500cal for women. Here is an example of how the classic workout cycle would look in your training schedule:

Monday: Low-carb day for men, 1500 cal for women and 1200 cal for men.

Tuesday: High carb day, 2000cals for men and 1500cals for women

Wednesday: Low-carb Day, 1500 Cal for Men / 1200 Cal for Women

Thursday: High-carb day. 2000cal for men, 1500cal for ladies

Friday: Low-carb day. 1500 cal for men, 1200 cal for women.

Saturday: High-carb day. 2000 Cal for men, 1500 Cal for women.

Sunday: Reward Day, 3000cal per man, 2500cal per woman

The Gym Buff's Pattern

This second sample is for dieters that prefer to work out three times per week. This pattern is often used by dieters who wish to gain muscle and reduce body fat. A low-carb diet will typically contain at most 150g carbohydrates, while high-carb diets will have at least 300g. This is an example:

Monday: A scheduled workout for the upper body. (High-carb day)

- Tuesday - Scheduled to do interval sprints. (Low-carb day)

- Wednesday: No training. (Low-carb day)

Thursday: Workout for lower body muscles (High-carb day)

Friday: Cardio exercises are scheduled. (Low-carb day)

Saturday: A complete body workout scheduled. (High-carb day)

Sunday: Training is not required. (Low-carb day)

The One No Carb Day - Pattern

Another way to do this is to add a no carb day to the cycle. A no-carb diet day is one in which the dieter is limited to taking any form of carbs. No-carb day can be extremely challenging because the daily allowance of carbohydrates should not exceed 30g. This could cause weakness if your body hasn't adjusted yet to the diet. But people who can cope well during low-carb meals have a greater chance of being able to withstand the no carb day.

The typical no-carb day is when the dieter will be taking a day off from their training. Even light exercises may not be possible on this cycle day. However, it will always depend how the dieter handles these situations. You should pace yourself during no-carb diet days.

It doesn't matter which diet the dieter follows, there is a general carbohydrate intake that everyone should follow. These are the grams of carbohydrates for each of the three types.

Day Carbohydrates Protein Fats

High-Carb Day 2g-2.5% Per Pound Weight

Low-Carb Day 1.5g/pound of Weight 1g-1.2g/pound 0.2g/pound

No-Carb Day, 0.5g/pound or 30g/day 1.5g/pound 0.35g-0.8g/pound

The Muscle Building Pattern

Another way to encourage lean muscle growth is through a pattern. A person will be required to eat low-carb for five days. Then, they will need to eat high-carb food on the next day. This pattern should not be used if you're training for a bodybuilding or sporting event. However, it can be useful if your tolerance is high and you have more carbs to build muscle mass faster. This is an example schedule for the pattern.

Monday: Low carb day (90g of carbs): Half the carbohydrates should be from fruits and vegetables, while half should come before or after exercise.

Tuesday: Tuesday is a low-carb day, with 90g of carbohydrates. You can divide all these carbs into portions of fruits or vegetables throughout the day.

Wednesday: Low-carb Day (90g Carbohydrates: All should be in some form sugar prior to and after working out).

Thursday: Low carb day (90g of carbs). All these should be used to make a serving of fruits and veggies throughout the day.

Friday: Low-carb Day (90g carbs): Half should come form fruits and vegetables, the other half should come in the form of sugar.

Saturday: High carb day (360g of carbohydrates): 100g should come primarily from fruits, vegetables, and 100g must be from some form sugar.

Sunday: Reward Day (720g of Carbohydrates: 120g should be fruits and vegetables, 100g should come from sugar, and the rest should go throughout the day.

Fat Trimming Pattern

Finally, this combination introduces a full-day fast and normal carb cycling days. A full day fast requires that a person eat absolutely nothing and does not work out. This program is intended to help you lose weight and tone your muscles. Here's an example of a workout program that uses this pattern.

MONDAY: TUESDAY WEDNESDAY TODAY FRIDAY SATURDAYSUNDAY

Activity Exercise Full-body and lower body workout Muscle builder Workout intervals to fat loss Muscle Muscle building Rest day Workout or rest day

Cycle High-carb diet Moderate carb day Low carb day Modate-carbday Full day fast Low -carbday

Carbohydrates 1.5g to 2.5g a pound of body 1.5g a pound of body 0.5g a pound 1,5g g a pound weight 1.5g g a pound weight 1.5g g a pound weight None 0.5g g g pound weight

Here's what you should keep in mind

It is important to remember that when choosing a carb-cycling pattern, one must consider his training and activities in order to get the most from the plan. For maximum muscle development, allocate high-carb meals to days that you have a schedule workout. Dedicate low-carb meals for days that you have more demanding activities.

You can expect changes to your body within one week. After two weeks, you will see the results no matter what type of carb cycling you are on. A carb cycling program should last for about 12 weeks. However this program can also be used for long-term weight loss, health maintenance, fitness, weight loss and bodybuilding.

In the next chapter I will talk about the details of carb cycling. This chapter will cover more details about carb cycling including ketosis (glycemic index), carb loading, and muscle development.

Chapter 14: The Nuances Of Carb Cycling

Carb Loading or Carb Cycling

For athletes and bodybuilders, it is essential to learn how to load carbohydrates correctly. Carb loading is an essential part of any bodybuilder or athlete's preparation for a sporting, or bodybuilding event. Carbohydrate loading is a way for athletes and bodybuilders to ensure their bodies are in top form before the competition.

Carb loading requires preparation. This is because it takes time for the body's to absorb and adjust. To get the best results, carb loading must be prepared for at least three days.

There is no need to change your diet if you're currently on a carb cycle diet. Simply take a week of your normal schedule and plan a six day carb loading prep. Here's a sample of carb loading during carb cycling.

Day 1 Day 2 Day 3, Day 4 Day 5, Day 6

Calories 1570cal 1400cal 1490cal 2200cal 3200cal 2200cal 3200cal 5200cal 6200cal 7200cal 8200cal 9200cal 1080cal

Carbohydrates   60g-60g
50g330g330g330g330g330g330g330g330g330g3
30g330g330g330g330g333g330g330g330g3
30g330g330g330g330g330g330g330g330g330g3
30g335g

Proteins 125g 125g 125g 190g 190g 190g

Fats 55g 55g 55g 85g 85g 85g

As the table shows, carb cycling is not a complete solution. You can still consume carbohydrates.

In this example, you will remove a week of your normal routine and change it to add carbs. In this case, the person was assigned three consecutive low carb days. Three high-carb days were followed by three more. The low-carb days prepare your body by removing excess fats. It is possible to still work out during this period, but it is essential to consume carbohydrates in some form of sugar prior to and after exercise to ensure you have enough energy for your muscles.

As the three-day carb loading day approaches, your body will be less hungry for carbohydrates and more open to receiving nutrients.

1. Your main goal on your first day carb loading is to get you back to your workout. During this time your muscles will crave all the carbohydrates you consume.

2. To get rid of that gloomy look you might have suffered from the low-carb three-day diet, you'll be eating high-carb meals on the second high carb day. This is the point when your muscles look fuller or more enlarged.

3. Last but not least, your body's carbohydrate intake should remain within normal limits on the final day of carb loading. This is the day your body achieves its most vibrant, powerful, lean, muscular, and energetic form.

Conclusion: To help your body reach its best form, carb loading is an important practice for athletes and bodybuilders. Because it works in the same way as a high-carb diet, you can use this diet for optimal carb loading.

Carb Cycling, Ketosis

For most people, losing excess fat can be difficult even for those who go to the fitness center regularly. A low-carb diet could solve this problem. There is the possibility of losing significant weight on this low-carb diet. This is because a person can lose not only excess weight but also water and muscle.

Carb cycling is a way to prevent weight loss that's not planned. It helps the body concentrate on burning fats and only fats throughout the entire duration of the program. This is why bodybuilders choose carb cycling over other diets. You can gain or maintain muscle mass and lose unwanted fats by carb cycling. This diet can also offset many of the adverse effects of low carb diets.

Ketosis, which is described above, is when the body searches for another source of energy. To reach this state, the body must exhaust its carbohydrate reserves. To lose weight, many people turn to low-carb diets. While it helps dieters lose weight fast, it can also make it difficult for them to stay motivated to do their workouts. After the body adjusts to ketosis the dieter may hit a wall, and then he'll have to start over.

To maintain ketosis, the main goal of carb cycling diet is to lose weight continuously without reaching a plateau. Because carb cycling involves a constant supply of carbohydrates, the process for ketosis is never ending and the body won't get used to it.

You must follow your carb cycling and nutrient intake every day to ensure that the body can go into ketosis. If there are too few carbs in the body, it may have difficulty getting into ketosis. This can lead to weight gain.

Conclusion: The body can stay healthy by consuming carb cycling while also losing excess body fats. Carb cycling aids the body get into ketosis. Ketosis assists in weight loss. Carb cycling helps ensure that the body doesn't lose its ability for fat burning by not acclimatizing to ketosis.

Carb Cycling, Glycemic Index of Foods

Carb cycling is an approach to reducing excess fat while training. It involves changing the amount of carbs a person consumes per day. It is helpful to understand the glycemic value of food in order to plan meals for optimal weight loss and muscle gain.

The glycemic indicator is a numerical representation of how carbohydrates impact blood sugar levels within 3 hours of eating. Carb foods that have high glycemic scores are often processed carb foods such as baked goods and white foods. Carb foods with low Glycemic Index are carb foods rich in fibre such as vegetables and fruits. Glycemic index usually refers to carbohydrates as this nutrient has a greater impact on blood sugar levels.

Glycemic index can be used for carb cycling to determine meal plans. When choosing foods for a carb cycling diet, there are three types of glycemic food ratings. These are:

Low GI food: Foods with a glycemic index of less than 50. Whole grain pita bread, whole grains, oatmeal, green leafy vegetable, natural fruit juices, eggs and shellfish are just a few examples.

Moderate GI food: Foods with 50 to 70 glycemicindex values. These foods include rice (baked beans), beet, cheese and beet.

High GI foods: Foods that have a 70+ glycemic score. This includes white bread, French toast, English muffins.

Conclusion: Carb cycling doesn't seem to be affected by food's glycemic content. It is a good idea to take this into account when you are choosing what foods to include in your meal plans. It is possible to create a healthier plan for carb cycle by combining your knowledge about nutrient values and information on glycemic.

Muscle Building, Carb Cycling

Bodybuilders build muscles by eating more and lifting weights. Once they have attained their desired muscle size, they begin a restricted diet program to get rid of any excess fats. You can build muscles with carb cycling without having to store much body fat

Carb cycling is a method of building muscle and a lean body. It involves learning how to use alternating cycles for building and cutting. To replenish the body's glycogen stores, and to maintain muscle growth, high-carb days are when a person will load carbohydrates into his body. Low-carb days will result in the body going into ketosis to burn extra fats. It is important to maintain a lean body and maintain muscle mass.

Bodybuilders eat only carbohydrates in sugar form during low carb days. They also take it before and afterwards a workout. This amounts to 0.5g for every pound of body weight. These days have two main goals: to reduce carb so the body burns excess fats, and to use sugars in order to drive nutrients and amino acids into the muscles.

To prevent the body's metabolism from stalling, it is important to increase the carbohydrate intake. This can help to prevent muscle loss. This day's carb intake should not exceed 2g per pound. As a result of the carb loading from the day before, bodybuilders tend to train large muscle groups the following a high-carb meal.

Rewards days are also important in order to build muscle. You will feel more energetic for your workouts at the gym when you have reward days. Your body will replenish its glycogen stores. This type of day will also boost your metabolism, which can help you lose more fat during low-carb diet days. For optimal muscle building, nutritional supplements are also administered to the muscles. Bodybuilders consume at minimum 4g of carbs per pound.

Conclusion: While carb cycling is not recommended for building or maintaining muscle mass, it is possible to do so. The diet can help build muscle and tone muscles as long the individual is mindful of their carb intake and follows a workout program.

Chapter 15: Getting Past The Fat Burning Plateau
You may notice a slowing down in your fat-burning efforts, even if you keep working hard at the gym. If this is not addressed, you will continue to work out for weeks but still see no progress.

A lot of people experience the feeling of hitting a wall while working out or dieting. As someone reaches his ideal body weight, their bodies will resist change and thus the fat-burning plateau. This concept is very simple. Because your body is leaner, you will burn less extra fat. This will result in your weight loss progress slowing down, and eventually stopping once your body has adjusted to your exercise and diet plan.

Low-carb diets will require you to cut down on your carb intake for a time. This will lead to weight loss and significant body fat reduction. It is important to remember that the longer a person is deficient in carbohydrates, the slower they will lose weight and reach a plateau in their metabolism. Once carbohydrates have been reintroduced to the body, it will then go into rebound mode which will make it difficult to lose weight.

Carb cycling makes it easy to lose weight without worrying about reaching a plateau. Carbohydrate cycling is a way to ensure that your body has enough carbohydrate supply to not slow down your metabolism. Low-carb days allow the body to enter a state that catabolic fat burners, which allows the body to burn unwanted body fats for the duration of the diet. The high-carb days increase metabolism and help the body burn more fats than low-carb.

The body keeps track of the nutrients it is receiving through carb cycling. This prevents it going into a metabolic decline that often occurs with linear diets. Another way to overcome the plateau is to eat a high-carbohydrate diet for a week every three weeks. Not only will it trick your metabolism, but your body will also be better equipped to absorb and use these nutrients. Implementing regular changes to your eating habits will ensure that you don't hit a wall in your fitness program.

Next chapter will cover healthy food sources and fats. I also include starter meal plans to show you how a day with no, low, and high carbohydrate options looks in terms of food. These meal plans can be used as a starting point for your diet or as a guideline for creating your own meal plan.

Chapter 16: Sample Meal Plans For Carb Cycling

There are two kinds of carbohydrates you can get in food: the good carbs as well as the bad carbs. Good carbs are foods that help to burn fats. Bad carbohydrates, on the other hand, are foods that make your body store more fat. I've listed different carb-loaded food and their respective good or bad carbs to help you choose the right source of carbohydrates.

Sources for Good Carbohydrates

- Sweet Potato

Brown Rice

Corn

Peas

- Beans

Oatmeal

- Whole wheat Pasta

Rice

Whole Grain Bread

Berries

- Green vegetables

- Fresh fruits

- Skimmed milk

Non-fat dairy product

Bad Carbohydrates Sources

Pastries

- Desserts

- Pizza

- Instant Oatmeal/Flavoured Oatmeal

- Ice cream

Fried foods

- Chocolates

- Candies

Soda

- Sweetened juices

Bacon

- Sausage

Chips

- Burgers and hotdogs

- Sweetened breakfast cereals

Here's a list that includes food you can include in your meal plans for low-, moderate-, and high carb days.

No or very low carbohydrate foods:

- Water

Turkey

- Cornish hen

Goose

- The Pheasant

- Quail

- Ostrich

- Chicken

Duck

Beef

- Lamb

Pork

Veal

- Venison

- Cod

Flounder

- Sole

Haddock

Halibut

Sardine

- Swordfish

- Tuna

Trout

Salmon

Lobster

- Shrimp

Squid

- Herring

Clams

Crabmeat

Olive oil

- Sunflower oil

Safflower oil

Corn oil

- Soybean oil

Canola oil

Peanut oil

- Sesame oil

- Walnut oil

Grape seed oil

Coconut oil

- Black coffee

Butter

Margarine

- Dillweed

- Mayonnaise

- Chives

- Vinegar

Alfalfa sprouts

Bok Choy

Radishes

- Lettuce

- Cheese (Parmesan, Camembert, Cheddar, Swiss, Provolone, Mozzarella, Blue Cheese, Cow, Sheep, Goat, Feta, Gouda)

Salami

- Eggs: Devilled, Fried (Har-Boiled), Omelettes; Poached.

Mustard

- Sour cream

- Tea

- Spinach

- Whipped cream

- Sausage

- Green pepper

Broccoli

- Cream cheese

Parsley

Cauliflower

- Tomatoes

- Escarole

- Fennel

Jicama

- Iceberg lettuce

Radicchio

- Romaine lettuce

Basil

- Cayenne pepper

Dill

Garlic

- Ginger

Oregano

Rosemary

Sage

Tarragon

- Daikon

Low-Carb Foods

Mussels

Bacon

Ham

Oyster

- Artichoke

- Artichoke hearts

Bamboo shoots

Broccoflower

- Brussels sprouts

Eggplants

- Green string beans

Hearts of palm

Kale

- Kohlrabi

- Leeks

Okra

- Green olives

- Black olives

- Onion

Pumpkin

Rhubarb

- Sauerkraut

- Snowpeas in pod

- Snappeas in a capsule

- Spaghetti squash

- Summer squash

- Turnips

- Water chestnuts

- Zucchini

- Chrysanthemum Leaves

- Endive

- Beet greens

Chicory greens

- Watercress

- New Zealand spinach

- Mustard spinach

- Nopales

Celery

- Collards

- Spinach

- Peeled cucumber

- Mustard greens

- Green leaf salad lettuce

Asparagus

Radishes

- Celtuce

- Chinese cabbage

- Arugula

- Zucchini

- Swiss chard

- Yellow summer squash

- White mushrooms

- Taro shoots

- Portabella mushrooms

- Avocados

- Chayote

- Starfruit

Blackberries

Raspberries

- Strawberries

- Rose-apple

- Gooseberries

- Pickly pears

- Peeled Lemons

- West Indian cherry

- Oheloberries

- Watermelon

- White grapefruit

- Cranberries

- Limes

- Peaches

Mulberries

- Honeydew melon

Cloudberries

Pomelo

- Huckleberries

- Nectarines

Guavas

- Corn bread

- Corn tortillas

Waffles

Popcorn

Saltine crackers

- Dried prunes

Orange

- Kiwi

- Cantaloupe

Cream of wheat

Hummus

- Dried cornmeal

- Red and pink grapefruit

High-Carb Foods

- Bagel

Pita bread

- Muffin

Pancakes

- Hamburger bun

- Croissants

- White bread

- Baked potato

- Squash

- Raisins

Dried apricot

- Bananas

Apples

- Pears

- Pineapples

- Fruit yoghurt

- Rice milk

Lima beans

- Garbanzo beans

- Kidney beans

- Lentils

Apple crispies

Brownies

- Danish

Granola

- Jellied cranberry sauce

Pudding

- Sherbet

- Sorbet

To prepare a better meal plan, you must know where to find your carbs. Be sure to balance all your nutrients throughout the day. Take for instance, if your day is low in carbs or zero, you should increase your intake of proteins and fats. On a high carb day, you should reduce your fat intake. These are the best fats and proteins that will help you get through low-carb days.

Sources of proteins:

- Chicken breast

Turkey breast

- Tuna

Salmon

Halibut

- Mozzarella cheese

Veal

Tofu

Pork chops

- Shellfish

- Mature soybeans

Yoghurt

- Milk

- Soy milk

- Pumpkin seeds

- Squash seeds

- Watermelon seeds

- Peanuts

Almonds

- Lean beef

- Cottage cheese

Quinoa

Dried beans

- Seitan

Eggs

Sources of Fats

Peanut butter

Flax oil

Heavy whipping Cream

- Mayonnaise

- Hemp oil

- Avocados

Butter

Eggs

Coconut oil

Bacon

- Sour cream

Ground beef up to 70%

- Cheddar cheese

Coconut

- Dark chocolate

- Cream cheese

- Fish oil

Olive oil

Each person has a unique body type and goals. Carb cycling is a flexible lifestyle. I didn't include a recommendation for nutrient intake. It is best to use it when you are active in your exercise program. You can use this template as a starting point and modify it as you need.

- PROTEIN. Because protein plays a crucial role in this diet, one must consume at most 1/6 (assuming six meals per daily) of the total daily requirements regardless of whether it is low-carb or higher-carb. The average dieter consumes 1.2g to 2.g protein per pound of his weight on low-carb days, but this can be adjusted according to his fitness goal. If a male weighs 200lbs and wants to consume 1g protein per pound, then he should eat 33g per meal (assuming six meals per days).

FATS: As fat is essential as an energy source, it is vital that the program is maintained and monitored. Remember that fat is an energy source. If you are low on carbs, it's a good idea to consume more. When you are high in carbs, it won't be as important.

CARBOHYDRATES. Because there are two to three different days for carbohydrate manipulation, dieters should be able to calculate the ratio of carbohydrate intake to calories and fats. Below is a chart displaying the ratios of carbohydrate intake to protein, fats, or carbohydrates for both low- and higher-carb days.

FOR MEN

Day Protein Fats Carbohydrates

High-Carb 1.7g 0.6g 1.7g

Low-Carb 1.5g 0.8g 0.9g

FOR WOMEN

Day Protein Fats Carbohydrates

High-Carb 1.4g 0.3g 1.4g

Low-Carb 1.2g 0.5g 0.6g

This chart contains the recommended levels and proportions of protein and fat during carb cycling. These can be modified to suit your specific goals but you should keep the ratios consistent to maximize effect. You can use the chart to calculate how much of each of these nutrients you should take daily by multiplying your body weight by those shown. To calculate the amount of calories one would receive for each macronutrient you will need to multiply your body weight by the value on the chart.

Supplements can be incorporated into your diet plan without fear. This dietary plan can be simplified by using protein shakes and other nutrient supplement like fish oil capsules. You can save time and money by using these supplements to simplify your meal plans. Supplements are a good way to get the nutrition you need, especially if there isn't any available food.

Junk food should not be considered as a food source. There is no set rule regarding junk food and carb cycling. However, it is better to avoid it as it could defeat the purpose for your diet.

You can download sample meal plans for a few days to help you get started with your diet. This is a sample meal plan that you can use as a guideline, or modify to suit your tastes or what food you have in your kitchen. You are good to go, as long you don't alter the carb count (e.g. when you choose another food).

No Carb Day Menu Plan #1: Calories - 1350cal Proteins, 135g Fats, 75g Carbohydrates and 30g

Breakfast: 2 boiled eggs, a cup tea or coffee and a cup.

100g leg Ham as a snack

Lunch: Barbecue chicken served with no stuffing

100g of shaved ham.

- Dinner - Barbecue, grilled fish.

No Carb Day 2: Calories: 885cal Proteins : 85g Fats : 50g Carbohydrates : 15g

- Breakfast: 2 scrambled or brewed eggs, a cup tea or coffee.

Snack: Egg Salad with Leafy Greens

- Lunch: Vegetable Salad with Cheese and Mayonnaise

Snacks: Two to three cheese slices

- Dinner: Grilled steak, green leafy vegetable.

Low Carb Day Meal Plans #1: Calories - 1645cal Proteins - 120g Fats - 85g Carbohydrates : 100g

Breakfast: A portion of vegetable salad with low calorie dressing and four eggs poached (fried), or scrambled.

Snack: 2 scoops Protein Powder mixed with water. Add a few handfuls of baby carrots or uncooked mixed nuts.

- Lunch: Salad with meats and vegetables

Snack: 2 scoops Protein Powder mixed with water. Several handfuls baby carrots and uncooked mixed Nuts. This meal is optional.

- Dinner: Beef Burger With Coconut and Cauliflower Massh

Low Carb Day Meal Plans #2: Calories 60g Proteins: 60g fats; 75g Carbohydrates 95g

Breakfast: Almond Fruit Salad and Citrus Salad

- Snack: A piece of apple and one bar Eat Natural

- Lunch: Quinoa Salad

Snack: A banana with a handful walnuts

- Dinner: Ginger Chicken

2 pieces of oatcakes as a snack

Low Carb Day Food Plan #3: Calories - 2025cal Proteins - 50g Fats - 95g Carbohydrates : 265g

Breakfast: 2 wholemeal pita bread slices with butter and 2 eggs boiled

Snacks: An apple or a pear.

- Lunch: Tuna and Avocado Mash

Snack: Peach, 4 pieces of oatcakes (cucumber and cottage cheese toppings)

- Dinner - Salmon Ratatouille

- Snack: One banana.

Low Carb Day Meal plan #4: Calories - 1995cal Proteins 120g Fats 95g Carbohydrates 170g

Breakfast: Omelette with chopped Ham and 1/3 of a cup of Oatmeal

Snack - A glass of protein powder.

- Lunch: Baked tuna, with a cup of green leafy veggies like spinach, green beans, and broccoli.

- Snack: A protein bar and carrot sticks.

- Dinner - Grilled chicken breasts served with vegetable salad and oil and vinegar dressing

Low Carb Day Menu Plan #5 - Calories: 1090 Cal Proteins: 45g Fatty Acids: 45g Carbohydrates. 140g

- Breakfast - Apple and Seed Muesli

Snack: One banana with a few nuts.

Lunch: Pita bread, tuna, avocado, and lowfat cottage cheese.

- Snack: A pear.

- Dinner - Lime Salmon Steak

Low Carb Day Menu Plan #6 - Calories: 1015cal Proteins, 70g Fats, 45g Carbohydrates and 85g

Breakfast: Tortillas without carbs

Snacks: An apple and some pumpkin seeds.

Salmon Salad

- Snack: One nectarine.

- Dinner: Grilled Turkey Breast With Mixed Vegetables

High Carb Day Plan #1: Calories - 2395cal Proteins - 165g Fats - 90g Carbohydrates. 240g

Breakfast: 1/2 cup oatmeal mixed with a handful fro frozen berries and three whole eggs The eggs can be poached or scrambled or fried.

Snack: 2 scoops Protein Powder mixed with water, 1 Banana, and several handfuls Uncooked Mixed Nuts.

- Lunch: A large sandwich made with whole grain bread that includes lots of meats and vegetables. A burrito made of whole wheat tortilla may be used in place of whole-grain bread.

Snack: 2 scoops Protein Powder mixed with water, 1 Banana, and several handfuls Uncooked Mixed Nuts. This meal is optional.

- Dinner: Healthy Pesto Chicken Pizza

#2: High Carb Day Meal Plans: Calories: 2110cal Proteins, 85g Fats, 65g Carbohydrates and 300g

Breakfast: Oatmeal with frozen Summer berries and sunflower seed, along with a pot of yoghurt.

- Snack: A peach.

Lunch: A baked potato served with hummus and mixed salad leaves, with tomatoes, cucumbers, red pepper, and banana.

Snack: An apple with a piece of Eat Natural.

- Dinner - Grilled cod fillet, boiled new potatoes and carrots, with garden peas and coriander.

- Snack: 3 pieces oatcakes

#3 High Carb Day Dinner Plan: Calories : 3310cal Proteins : 175g Fatty Acids : 80g Carbohydrates. 510g

Breakfast: Six ounces of skimmilk, an omelette and half cup of oatmeal.

Snack: Half cup of yoghurt with 4 to 5 strawberries

Lunch: Half a cup of brown Rice and half of a chicken breast.

Snack: An apple with a protein bar.

- Dinner - Grilled steak with two cups vegetable soup, including spinach, cucumber, green onions or radishes

#4 High Carb Day Menu Plan: Calories, 1940cal Proteins and 145g Fats. 25g Carbohydrates. 300g

Breakfast: One egg (fried or boiled), 6 oz skimmilk and one banana

Snack: 2 scoops Protein Powder mixed with water and 4-5 slices of Peach.

Lunch: Grilled tuna and sweet potato with a cup each of spinach, green bean, or asparagus.

- Snacks include canned tuna, whole grains bread, and celery or carrot sticks.

- Dinner: Chicken breasts or turkey served with vegetable salad and oil and vinegar dressing.

Carb cycling requires you to consume five meals per days. This is to ensure your body remains healthy over the course of the diet. You won't feel deprived of food because you will be eating at minimum five times per day.

Remember to spread your meals evenly throughout your day so that you can properly distribute the nutrients needed to keep your body fit and healthy during carb cycling. Make sure you never eat less that three hours after your last meal. Remember to hydrate your body. Water should be at least 1 gallon per day. This will allow you to replenish the water you lost from your diet and exercise. Water can provide you with a feeling of fullness and help you avoid hunger pangs during low carb days.

BREAKFAST RECIPES

Mango Coconut Yogurt Bowl

Low-Carb

Serves 2. Prep time: 5 mins

Ingredients

1/4 cup unsweetened, shredded coconut

1/2 cup light coconut milk

2 cups plain nonfat Greek yogurt

1 cup chopped mango, fresh or frozen

Instructions

In a small bowl combine the yogurt, coconut milk and sugar until well blended. Add mango and shredded chocolate to the bowl before serving.

Per serving (1 bowl): Fat: 10g Protein: 27g Fiber: 2g Carbohydrates : 24g Calories: 287

Apple Pie Overnight Oats

High-Carb

Serves 2 Prep Time: 10 Mins, Plus Soaking Overnight

Ingredients

 1 scoop Vanilla whey Protein Powder

 1 1/2 cups rolled Oats

1/4 teaspoon groundnutmeg

 1 teaspoon ground Cinnamon

1/4 teaspoon salt

 2 Tablespoons Maple Syrup

 14 teaspoon ground ginger

1/8 teaspoon allspice

1/4 cup nonfat milk

2/3 cup plain nonfat Greek yogurt

1/2 apple, diced

Instructions

1. Divide the oats powder, protein powder and ginger evenly between two single serve containers. Combine with a spoon.

2. Divide the Greek Yogurt, Maple Syrup, and Milk between the two containers. Mix thoroughly.

3. In each container, add half the diced apple. Cover the container and put in the fridge overnight.

Serving: (1 Cup) Calories, Fat, and Protein: 377. Fiber: 8g. Carbohydrates: 61g.

Low Carb Creamy Egg Cups with Bacon & Egg
Yield: 12

Prep time for the exam: 10 minutes

Cook time: 22 minutes

Total time: 32 Mins

Ingredients

cooking spray

12 large eggs

1/2 cup parmesan cheese

12 bacon slices

Black pepper

Garlic salt

1 Tablespoon fresh chives (chopped).

Instructions

1. Preheat oven to 400F

2. Bake the bacon for 8-9 minutes on a baking pan in the centre of the oven, depending upon the thickness. Bake the bacon until it's lightly browned and still very flexible. Let it cool.

3. Grease a muffin tin of standard size.

4. Each slice of bacon should always be wrapped in a muffin pan. Make sure to wrap as much bacon as possible in muffin cups.

5. Cover each cup with a little bit of parmesan cheese.

6. Crack an egg into each cup.

7. Sprinkle fresh chives on top.

8. Bake the eggs for 10-12 minutes on the center rack of the oven or until they are cooked to your liking. The egg should not be overcooked.

9. Sprinkle with garlic salt

10. Sprinkle with salt.

11. Serve immediately, and enjoy!

Keto Sausage Balls Recipe, Low Carb

Prep Time: 15 Minutes

Cook Time: 17 Minutes

Total Time: 32 minutes

Servings: 36 Calories: 89kcal

Ingredients

 2 tablespoons full-fat cream

 1/3 cup coconut oil

4 1/2 tbsp chilled melted butter

1 lb Breakfast drained Brown Sausage (Can be used hot or cold)

4 eggs

2 cups sharp shredded cheddar cheese shredded

1/4 teaspoon salt

14 teaspoon baking powder

Instructions

1. Preheat the oven to 325 degrees.

2. Butter a cookie sheet.

3. Blend the cooled butter with salt, sour milk, and eggs. Finally, whisk together. Let the molten butter cool for around 10 minutes in the fridge.

4. Add coconut flour and baking soda to the mixture. Mix well until well combined

5. Add the sausage (browned and drained).

6. Stir in the cheese. Finally, place the batter into the refrigerator for ten minutes. The batter should remain warm for at least 10 minutes. If it is not, refrigerate for a longer time. This is

necessary to prevent sausage balls from drying out when baking. They don't form perfectly formed balls when baked, they more resemble puffs.

7. Drop batter by carefully packing spoonfuls on greased cookie sheets. I made 36.

8. Bake for between 14-18 minutes or until edges are slightly brown.

Oven-Baked Easter Eggs in A Muffin Tin

Prep time: 1 min

Cook Time: 15 Minutes

Total time: 16 minutes

Servings: 12 eggs

Calories: 62kcal

Ingredients

Nonstick Cooking Spray

Salt and pepper to suit your tastes

1 Dozen Eggs

Instructions

1. Preheat oven to 350F

2. In a muffin pan, place the eggs. Add a little salt and pepper to the eggs.

3. Bake at 350°F for 15 minutes.

4. Let cool in the refrigerator. Take out each egg with a spoon. Transfer them to a container. The eggs can be kept in the fridge up to four days.

Nutrition

Fat: 4g

Sausage Egg Muffins

Prep time: 15 mins

Cooking Time: 40 Minutes

Total Time: 55 minutes

Servings: 12 egg muffins Calories: 246kcal

Ingredients

3 tablespoons of coconut oil

1 lb sausage

3 tablespoons of ground golden flax

1/2 teaspoon salt

3 tablespoons almond flour

1 cup cheddar cheese

12 eggs

1/4 teaspoon pepper

1 teaspoon fresh rosemary chopped finely

Instructions

1. Preheat oven 400. Spray a 12-hole muffin mold with cooking spray. Spray both the sides and the top of the muffin pan with cooking spray.

2. Combine the sausage, ground flax, coconut flour and almond flour. Split the sausage into 12 pieces. Place each piece in a muffin tin. Gently crack an egg into each. Sprinkle with salt. Bake for 30 minutes.

3. Sprinkle the cheese and rosemary over the top. Bake for another 7-10 minutes or until the sausage has cooked thoroughly and the cheese is melted and bubbly.

Nutrition

Fat: 19g

90-Second Keto French Toast

Prep Time: 5 Mins

Cooking time: 10 minutes

Total time: 15 minutes

Course: Breakfast

Servings: 1 Calorie: 352kcal

Ingredients

 1 egg

 1 Tablespoon coconut flour

 1 tsp cream Cheese

 12 teaspoon of nutmeg

 1/4 tsp baking soda

 1 1/4 tbsp butter, melted

 1/4 teaspoon cinnamon

 For French Toast

1/4 teaspoon Lakanto Monkfruit Powdered Zucker

 1 egg

1 cup heavy whipping cream

Instructions

1. Make butter in a glass bowl.

2. Mix together the remaining ingredients until well combined.

3. Cook in the microwave at 90 secs

4. Take the microwave out and allow it to cool.

5. Divide the bread in half

6. To make the heavy whipping and 1 egg, place in a flat bowl. Stir well.

7. You can soak both sides in heavy whipping crème and in egg.

8. Place 1 tbsp butter on a frying plate and fry each side till crisp.

9. Sprinkle 1/4 teaspoon Lakanto sweetener.

Keto Low Carb Bagels Recipe Using Fathead Dough Gluten Free

Ingredients

2 large Egg (beaten)

2 1/2 cup shredded Mozzarella cheese

1 tablespoon Baking Powder

2 oz Cream cheese (cubed)

1 1/2 cups Wholesome Yum Blanched Almond Flaour

Instructions

1. Preheat oven to 400F. Bake on parchment paper.

2. Combine the almond flour, baking powder, and salt. Set aside.

3. In a large bowl combine the cubed cream and shredded mozzarella. Microwave for 2 minutes. Stir gently halfway through. At the end stir once more until all is well.

4. Stir together the flour mixture, eggs, and melted cheese. Make a dough by mixing the flour mixture with the eggs while it is still warm.

Although the dough may be sticky, continue to squeeze and knead it for about a minute. If the dough becomes sticky or too difficult to mix, or is still hard after a while, you can heat it up again in the microwave for 17-20 seconds. You can wash your hands with water after mixing the dough.

5. Split the dough into six equal-sized pieces. To make a bagel, roll each portion into a long log. Then press the ends together on the baking sheet. You can do the same with the rest of your dough.

6. Bake bagels in the oven for between 10 and 15 minutes or until golden brown.

Serving size: 1 bagel

Herb Baked Eggs

Serves: 4

Ingredients

1 teaspoon chopped oregano

1 clove garlic, minced

1 1/2 tablespoons parsley, minced

2 tablespoons grated parmesan cheese

1 teaspoon minced thyme leaf

1/4 cup heavy whipping cream

12 large eggs

2 tablespoons unsalted margarine

Salt and pepper to suit your taste

Toasted French Bread, for serving

Instructions:

1. Preheat the broiler for approximately 4 minutes

2. Place the oven rack approximately six inches below your heat.

3. Combine the garlic and oregano with the parsley, parsley, and thyme. Set aside. You should crack 3 eggs carefully in 4 small bowls. Take extra care not too break the yolks.

4. Four individual gratins should be placed on one baking sheet. Each dish should contain a half-tbsp butter and 1 tbsp cream. Bake the dish in the oven for 2-3 minutes or until hot. To make each

individual gratin, carefully pour 3 eggs into each dish. Next, sprinkle the herb mixture equally over each dish. Then sprinkle lightly with salt and pepper. Put the eggs back under the broiler and cook for another 4-6 mins until the whites are nearly cooked. If the eggs don't cook evenly, turn the baking sheet.

5. After taking the eggs out from the oven they will continue to cook. Allow the eggs to rest for one minute before serving hot with toasted bread.

Keto Berry Mug Cake

Nutritional content (per portion)

Net Carbohydrates: 4.4%

Protein: 12.1 grams

Fat: 28.5g

Calories: 344 kcal

Ingredients (one portion)

1 heaping tablespoon coconut oil

 2 heaping teaspoons almond flour

1 large egg

1/8 teaspoon baking soya

1/2 teaspoon sugar-free vanilla extract

1 tablespoon Erythritol, or Swerve

3-5 drops liquid Stevia

1 Tablespoon melted butter, extra-virgin Coconut oil

A few berries - can either be frozen, fresh, mixed, or preserved.

Instructions

1. Mix all dry ingredients into a mug. Combine. Add the egg to the mixture.

2. Use coconut oil and vanilla extract.

3. Mix the stevia with the mixture. Add berries (frozen, fresh or mixed).

4. Microwave for around 90 seconds on high

Keto Blueberry Pancakes Gluten-Free
Prep Time: 5 Mins

Cook Time: 15 Minutes

Total time: 20 minutes

Calories: 228kcal

Servings: 6

Ingredients

3 eggs, separately

3/4 cup almond meal

1/2 cup Oat Fiber

3/4 cup fresh blueberries

3/4 cup heavy whipping cream

1 teaspoon pure vanilla extract

2 teaspoons baking flour

2 tablespoons swerve confectioners/ powdered Erythritol

Avocado oil or coconut oil can be used for the pan.

Instructions

1. Separate the egg whites. With a hand mixer whip the egg yolks in a bowl until they reach soft peak.

2. In another bowl, mix the heavy cream with egg yolks, swerve, vanilla, and then transfer to a new bowl. Use a hand mixer to combine for around 2 minutes. Mix in the egg yolks.

3. In a separate bowl, combine the almond flour and baking powder in a large bowl. Mix the wet mixture into the dry ingredients. Stir until everything is well combined. The batter should not be too loose. You may add more heavy cream if you need.

4. Cook the pancake batter in coconut oil, avocado oil, clarified butter/ghee on low heat. Add 3-5 blueberries to each pancake.

5. You should cook them for a few minutes on each side on low heat.

Low Carb Pumpkin waffles

Prep Time: 5 Mins

Cook Time: 5 Minutes

Total time: 10 minutes

Total Carbohydrates: 7g

Net Carbs: 3g

Protein: 4 g

Servings: 8 quarters waffle

Ingredients

 1 teaspoon baking powder

 2 tsp pumpkin pie spice

 0.5 teaspoon xanthan Gum

1 cup almond meal

 2 tablespoons of low-carb granulated sweetener

 2 large eggs

1/4 cup pumpkin puree (60mls)

 1/4 cup water, 60mls

 0.5 teaspoon vanilla extract

Instructions

1. Combine all dry ingredients (e.g., almond flour, baking mix (not baking soda), xanthan Gum, low

carbgranulated sweetener, pumpkin pie spice) in a bowl. Use a spoon to combine everything.

2. Combine the dry ingredients (eggs, pumpkin puree, vanilla extract and water) in another bowl. Stir well until everything is combined.

3. Mix the wet ingredients and dry ingredients together until you have a smooth mixture.

4. Put half of the batter in the middle a hot, greased waffle-iron. Spread the batter out with a spatula. Depending upon the waffle maker, the amount of mixture you use will yield approximately four quarter-sized waffles.

5. Close the waffle iron and let it cook for a few minutes. Timing will depend on how hot the waffle iron is.

6. They will be soft when cooked but will harden once they cool. Due to the almond flour, the waffles won't turn out as crisp as traditional waffles.

7. Serve hot with low-carb maple pancake syrup.

Serving size 1/4 waffle

Baked Tomato Eggs

Prep Time: 10 Mins

Cooking time: 20-25 minutes

Total Time: 30-35 Minutes

Yield: 2-3 portions

Ingredients

Sea salt for taste

6 medium red tomatoes

6 large, pasture-raised eggs

black pepper to flavor

1 teaspoon flat leaf parsley chopped (optional).

Instructions

1. Take 1/4 off the tomato's top. Grab a grapefruit spoon and scrape out the inner membrane, seeds, and other parts until you only have the hollow shell. Do the same thing for the other tomatoes.

2. Place each cut tomato in a muffin tin or on a baking pan. One egg should be poured into each

cup. For a soft egg, bake at 350F for 18-20 mins. For a hard egg, bake at 350F for 23-25mins.

3. Let it cool.

4. Sprinkle with pepper, salt and chopped flatleafparsley.

5. Restricted leftovers can be kept in the fridge up to five days.

Baked Eggs In Avocado

Servings: 2

Ingredients

 2 ripe avocados

 1 tbsp minced chives

 1/8 tsp.

 4 fresh eggs

Instructions

1. Preheat oven to 425F

2. Split the avocados in two. You can remove the pit.

3. You will need to scoop out approximately 2 tbsp flesh from the middle of the avocado. Make sure the egg is big enough to fit in the middle.

4. Place the avocados in a small, but suitable baking bowl.

5. In the avocado halves, crack the four eggs. Allow the yolk to drip in first. Then add the eggwhites to fill the remainder of the avocado shell.

6. Place in the oven

7. Bake for 18-20mins. (Depending on the size and shape of the avocados or eggs, the cooking time may vary). It is vital that the egg whites are allowed to set for a sufficient time.

8. Remove from oven

9. Season the salad with chives, pepper, and whatever garnishes you prefer.

10. Serve and enjoy

Nutrition

Calories per serving: 449 kcal

Chicken And Apple Sausage

Yield: 4

Ingredients

2 large chicken breasts

1 Apple, peeled and finely diced

1 Tablespoon fresh Thyme leaves, finely chopped

1 Tablespoon fresh rosemary, finely chopped

3 Tablespoons fresh chopped parsley

2 teaspoons garlic oil

salt and pepper

Coconut oil to cook with

Instructions

1. Preheat oven to 425 degrees F.

2. Put 3 tablespoons of coconut oil in a pan. Once the apples are softened, cook them on medium heat for 6-8 mins.

3. Take it off the heat, and let it cool for 5 minutes.

4. Cook the chicken breast.

5. Mix the chicken meat, garlic powder, pepper, salt, and any remaining oil in the fryingpan.

6. Take 12 small patties of meat (1/2") and form them into thin patties.

7. Bake for 20 minutes.

8. Cool and place in the fridge or freezer.

9. Pan-fry the sausages for a few minutes in coconut oil if you prefer them to brown. You can also pan fry the raw sausages rather than baking them.

Baked Eggs in Ham Cups

Yield: 2 Serving Sizes: 1

Ingredients

 2 Eggs

 2 slices of Deli meat, ham

 1 teaspoon of cooking oil

 Cooking spray (optional)

Instructions

1. Preheat oven to 400F

2. Cook oil can be used to grease the Cupcake Pan. You can either spray it with cooking spray, or sprinkle some Coconut Oil over it.

3. Place 1 or 2 slices de ham in each muffin cup.

4. You don't have to scramble your eggs. Instead, crack one egg into a separate bowl. Beat it then pour it into the ham cups. This version cooks more quickly than the unscrambled.

5. If you prefer your eggs whole and not scrambled then crack the egg in the hamcup. Some eggs may be too big. You can make sure that you don't get any eggs in a mess by first breaking the eggs into a separate bowl, then pour the egg mixture into a ham cup.

6. Bake for 12-15 minutes. Depending upon how much you love eggs and the time it takes to bake, you have the option of extending or reducing baking time.

Nutrition Information:

Trans Fat: 0g

Mexican Breakfast Bowl

Ingredients

1/4 cup Cheddar Cheese

1/2 ripe avocado

2 large eggs

1 Tablespoon sour Cream

1 link chorizo (4 oz)

1/4 small tomato

Instructions

1. Over medium heat, cook the chorizo in a skillet.

2. Place the cookedchorizo on top of a piece paper towel.

3. You can also pour out some of these greases, leaving some behind to cook your eggs.

4. Mix two eggs in a medium skillet with chorizo oil and stir to combine. You can add milk to make it fluffier.

5. Once the eggs have been cooked, place them at the bottom of a bowl.

6. Spread the chorizo on top of the eggs. Add the avocado, tomato, cheese, sour milk, and cilantro.

7. Serve immediately, while warm.

LUNCH RECIPES

Avocado Bacon Crustless Quiche Recipe

Prep time: 10 min

Cook Time: 30 minutes

Total Time: 40 minutes

Servings: 6 Servings Calories = 176kcal

Ingredients

6 large eggs

1/4 cup 2% Milk or Your preferred milk/milk Alternative

1/4 teaspoon salt 1 cup chopped bacon (about 6 pieces)

1/4 teaspoon ground black Pepper

1/2 cup shredded mozzarella cheese

1 avocado peeled. Seeded. Chopbed.

Instructions

1. Preheat oven to 350F

2. Using a cooking spray, spray a standard pie plate.

3. In a medium bowl combine the milk and eggs with salt. Combine all ingredients in a bowl.

4. Add the bacon and avocado to the bowl. Stir it gently until it is well-mixed.

5. Put the egg mixture on the pie plate. To ensure the egg mixture is evenly distributed, use a spoon to push the avocado and bacon around.

6. Bake for 30 minutes. Rotate once halfway through.

7. Let the quiche cool completely before slicing.

Nutrition

Protein: 11.4g

Buffalo Chicken and Broccoli Bowls
Prep time: 10 mins

Cook Time: 20 minutes

Serving Size: 4

Ingredients

Cauliflower Rice

1 tbsp olive oil

1 head cauliflower

pepper

Salt

Broccoli & Buffalo Chicken

1 pound of chopped broccoli in small to medium florets

1 lb skinless and boneless chicken breast cut into bite-sized pieces

1/4 cup hot sauce

Optional:

2 tbsp butter

Pepper

Salt

Instructions

Cauliflower and Rice

1. Cut cauliflower into small to medium-sized cubes.

2. Take out any tough stems.

3. Work in batches. Place the florets on a food processor. Continue to process until the filling is complete. (Be sure to not go over halfway).

4. About 18 pulses should be enough to get the cauliflower looking like rice grains. Avoid over-processing or you'll end up with cauliflower mash.

5. Over medium heat, heat olive oil in a skillet or saute pan. Season the cauliflower with salt. Saute until tender 5-8 mins.

How to Make Buffalo Chicken & Broccoli

1. A skillet or sautepan that has a cover can be heated over medium-high heat. When the oil is heated, add the oil. Season with a small amount of salt. Turn the pieces over to brown one side, and then turn them over to brown the opposite side. Cook until no longer pink (4-5 minutes per side).

2. Cover the pan with broccoli once the chicken is cooked. Allow to steam for about 5-10 mins. To avoid the chicken getting too brown, you should stir the pan occasionally.

3. Make the buffalo sauce. Mix the butter and hot sauce in a small saucepan. Whisk to combine.

4. Spread the buffalo sauce on the broccoli and chicken. Stir gently to coat the sauce.

5. Serve over regular rice or cauliflower rice.

Grilled Salmon Kebabs

Prep Time: 15 mins

Cook Time: 10 mins

Total Time: 25 mins

Yield: 4 Servings

Ingredients

2 tablespoons chopped fresh oregano

2 teaspoons sesame oil

1/4 teaspoon crushed red chili flakes

1 teaspoon ground cumin

1 1/2 lb wild salmon skinless fillet, cut into 1-inch chunks

Olive oil cooking spray

2 lemons cut thinly into rounds

16 bamboo-skewers, soaked in 60 minute water

1 teaspoon kosher sodium

Instructions

1. Turn the heat up to medium.

2. Apply olive oil to the grates.

3. Mix together sesame seed, cumin and red pepper flake in a small bowl.

4. Place the spice mixture aside.

5. Make 8 kebabs by threading salmon and lemon slices onto 8 pairs each of parallel skewers.

6. Apply olive oil lightly to the fish.

7. Season the fish in kosher Salt and the reserved spice combination.

8. Grill the fish. Turn the fish occasionally until opaque. About 7 to 10 minutes.

Healthy Avocado Chicken Salad

Prep Time: 5 mins

Cooking time: 20 mins

Serves: 6

Ingredients

1 avocado

2 cups shredded Chicken

12 teaspoon garlic powder

1/2 teaspoon salt

1/2 teaspoon pepper

2 teaspoons lime juice

1 teaspoon fresh chopped cilantro

1/4 cup mayonnaise

1/4 cup plain Greek Yogurt

Instructions

1. Combine all ingredients together in a large bowl. To let flavors blend, cover with a lid.

2. Serve your favorite crackers or pita pockets on bread, or on a bed with lettuce.

Nutrition Information:

Calories 202kcal (10%) Protein: 13g (16%) Fat 15% 15g (23%) Cholesterol : 39mg (13%) Potassium : 281mg (12%) Calcium: 19mg (2%) Iron : 0.8% (4%)

Asian Edamame Salad, With Cilantro & Toasted Almonds

Prep Time: 15 mins

Total time: 15 mins

Serves: 4

Ingredients

3 cups shelled Edamame Beans, cooked and cooled

1 red bell Pepper, diced

1 orange bell pepper diced

12 cup freshly grated ginger

1 Cup shredded carrots

1/2 head purple/red carrot, shredded

2 tablespoons sesame oil

1/2 tbsp honey/agave syrup

1/4 cup reduced-sodium soy sauce or gluten-free soy sauce

2 cloves garlic, minced

1/4 cup toasted nuts

1/2 cup fresh chopped coriander

Instructions

1. Combine cabbage, diced bell and red peppers, carrots and edamame into a large bowl.

2. For your dressing, whisk together the sesame oils, ginger, honey, soya sauce, and garlic. Toss the dressing in the edamame mix and stir well.

3. Include cilantro.

4. Mix well and add the toasted almonds.

Crustless Spinach Bacon Quiche

Prep Time: 15 Minutes

Cook Time: 45 Minutes

Total Time: 1hr

Servings: 6

Calories: 327kcal

Ingredients

A 16-ounce bag freeze spinach. Thawed and squeezed dry.

1/3 pound cooked and chopped bacon

2 ounces minced onion or thinly chopped

6 large eggs

3/4 cup heavy whipping cream

1/4 teaspoon salt

1/4 tsp.

1 pinch nutmeg

8 ounces cheddar or Swiss cheese, grated

Instructions

1. The bacon should be cooked until crisp.

2. Grease a pie dish (8x8) or a glass dish (8x8). Preheat oven to 350F

3. Thaw the spinach. Let it air dry. Slice the onion thinly to make mince or halves. Grate cheese.

4. Mix all ingredients together in a large bowl. Use a hand mixer or a whisk to combine all the ingredients. Transfer to the prepared pan. Spread using a rubber spatula. Put in the middle of the oven. Cook for 40 mins.

5. Serve warm. Freeze for up 2 weeks or refrigerate up to 3 months.

6. Serves 6 at 4 net carbohydrates per person

Nutrition

Calories: 327kcal | Carbohydrates: 6.5g | Protein: 20g | Fat: 26g | Sodium: 780mg | Fiber: 2.5g

Bacon Lettuce Tomato Spring Rolls
Yields 6 servings

Preparation time: 15 mins

Cook time: 5 mins

Total time: 20 mins

Ingredients

Bacon Lettuce Tomato Spring Roll:

6 pieces bacon, cooked

1 medium tomato (seeded & sliced 1/4inches thin)

6-12 leaves fresh lettuce, cut or torn pieces

Fresh basil, mint, or any other herbs

12 avocado slices, optional

6 rice paper

Sesame-Soy Dipping Sauce:

1/4 cup chilled water

1/4 cup Soy Sauce

1 teaspoon Sesame Oil

1 teaspoon fresh Lime Juice

Instructions

Instructions for spring roll

1. Fill a large container with water. Heat the water by adding hot water. Warm water can be used to dampen each wrapper of rice paper. Take

care not to soak the rice papers too much. It will continue to absorb the hot water after being removed from the warm water.

2. Place rice papers on a plate. Add fillings once the paper absorbs water and becomes softer and pliable (usually 15-20 seconds, depending upon water temp. and wrappers).

3. Pick a rice paper wrapper. Layer tomatoes, lettuce, bacon and other fillings on the one-third portion of the ricepaper wrapper. Only one slice can be added to a spring roll. For extra flavor, two slices of bacon may be added to a spring roll.

4. You will need to roll the wrapper in a circular motion over the fillings. Continue rolling and tucking it with your fingers.

5. Serve immediately, wrap in plastic wrap and let cool for several hours.

Instructions for Sesame and Soy Dipping Sauce

1. Combine all ingredients in a small mason-jar.

2. Close the lid. Shake vigorously for 15-20 seconds or until everything is well combined.

Nutritional Information

Shawarma Chicken Bowls - Basil-Lemon Vinaigrette

Serves: 4

Ingredients

Chicken Shawarma:

1 lb free range organic chicken breast, cut in 3-inch strips

2 tbsp Lemon juice

3/4 tsp fine grain sea salt

2 tbsp olive oil

1 teaspoon curry Powder

3 minced garlic cloves

1/2 teaspoon ground cumin

1/4 tsp ground chiliander

Salad:

1 avocado, sliced

6 cups spring greens

2 handfuls of fresh basil leaves rubbed

1 cup cherry tomatoes, halved

Basil-Lemon Vinaigrette:

1/2 tsp fine grain sea salt

5 tbsp olive oil

2 large bunches of fresh basil leaves

1 clove garlic, mashed

2 tablespoons freshly squeezed lemon juice

Instructions

1. In a bowl, whisk together lemon juice and salt.

2. Combine marinade, chicken strips and ziploc bag.

3. Cover the meat with a plastic wrap or seal it and place in the refrigerator.

4. To prepare the meal, heat an oven-safe nonstick pan on medium heat.

5. You can add a small amount of olive oil to the chicken, and then cook it until it turns golden brown.

6. Start making the vinaigrette. Blend the garlic and lemon juice with the basil until smooth. Add the oil slowly to the mixture. Blend until the oil is well combined. When you are satisfied, turn off the heat and set aside.

7. Place the greens in an large bowl to make the salads. Toss in some salt and pepper. Serve the chicken over the basil, tomatoes, avocado.

8. Serve the bowl with the basil-lemon dressing.

9. Enjoy!

Nutrition facts

One serving provides 392 calories and 28 grams fat. It also contains 9 grams carbs and 27 grams protein.

Thai Stuffed Avocados

Serves: 2

Time: 10 Mins

Ingredients:

1/2 cup cream cheese

1 large avocado, a little firm but ripe

1/3 cup hummus

spicy sprouts

1 tbsp chili garlic sauce

sriracha sauce

roasted peanuts

Instructions

1. Mix the hummus and cream cheese in a large bowl. Add the chili garlic sauce.

2. The avocado should be cut in half. You can remove the pit. You can slice the avocado, but you should keep it in its skin. Use your knife to create a checkerboard pattern on the avocado so it is easy to scoop.

3. Spread a generous portion of the cream cheese mixture on each half of an avocado. Sprinkle with sprouts, peanuts, sriracha sauce, and garnish with the remaining cream cheese mixture. Enjoy immediately!

Buffalo Chicken Lettuce Wraps
Prep Time: 5 Mins

Cooking time: 15 minutes

Total time: 20 minutes

Ingredients

2 large breasts of chicken cooked and shredded

1/2 tbsp olive oil

1/2 cup Franks Red Hot Wing Sauce

2 tbsp butter

Fresh peppers to taste

1/2 teaspoon celery seeds

blue cheese crumbles

1 cup thinly sliced celery

2 heads (romaine or Iceberg) of lettuce, washed and dried.

ranch dressing

Instructions

1. Cook the chicken and shred it in a large pot.

2. Keep the heat on medium or low. Blend the olive oil and butter together. Continue stirring

until well combined. Then add the celery seed, hot-sauce, and pepper to taste. Reduce heat to low and gently stir in celery sliced thinly.

3. Make lettuce wraps by putting a teaspoonful of the chicken mixture into each lettuce leaf. Sprinkle with blue cheese crumbles. Drizzle with ranch dressing.

4. Serve!

Big Fat Nori Wraps

Prep Time 20 minutes

Cook Time: 1 minute

Ingredients (1 serving)

2 sheets nori seaweed

A small bowl of warm liquid

Fillings

1/3 cup baby spinach leaves

1 small carrot, shredded

1/4 English cucumber, cut into strips the same size as the nori sheets, and then cut into long thin pieces

1/4 cup thinly-sliced purple cabbage

4 shredded, or very thinly cut red radishes

1/4 cup sprouts (alfalfa/broccoli, sunflower/lunch, etc.) - homegrown and store-bought

1/4 avocado thinly sliced

Optional: chopped cilantro

For the spread of cilantro sunflower:

3/4 cup raw unsalted sunflower seeds

1/4 cup loosely packaged cilantro

1 clove minced garlic

1 teaspoon lime juice

1 Tablespoon minced fresh ginger

1 Tablespoon rice vinegar

1 teaspoon low sodium Tamari

Instructions

1. All ingredients for the sunflower spread form are to be combined in a food processer. It will not be smooth, but it is fine.

2. Assemble all fillings following the instructions.

3. Lay the first nori sheets on a sushi roll mat. Begin by spreading a thin layer sunflower along the edge of your nori sheet. Continue to spread the sunflower from left and right. (Note - You want a rectangle shape that covers about 1" of the sheet and is about 1/2cm high.

4. In that order, arrange some of the spinach leaves on the sunflower spread. Add a few long pieces of cucumber, purple carrot, carrot, radish or sprouts to the mix.

5. Grab the nori sheets and sushi mat ends closest to you, and then roll them away.

6. The mat should be tightened by a slight tug when you reach the point that the nori mat and mat are above the fillings. Refrain from tugging on seaweed. This will cause it to tear.

7. Continue rolling away the nori sheet, letting it fall to the side.

8. Warm water can be applied to the nori sheets with your fingers after you get to its edge. For sealing the wrap, roll it up and place seam side down on a plate.

9. Split the wrap in half. Trim the extra nori at ends and fold it under. Continue the process with the remaining nori sheets and fillings.

10. You can also enjoy it with low-sodium, tamari as a dip.

Stir Fry with Keto Asian Cabbage

Ingredients

1 lb green cauliflower

2 oz. Butter, butter, or coconut oil

1 teaspoon salt

1 teaspoon onion paste

1/4 teaspoon ground Black Pepper

1 Tablespoon white wine vinegar

2 garlic cloves, minced

1 teaspoon Chili Flakes

2 tablespoons minced or grated fresh ginger

1 1/4 Lbs ground beef/ground turkey

3 (1 1/2 oz.) Calamari, cut in 1/2" (1.5 cm), slices

1 tablespoon sesame oil

1 cup mayonnaise or vegan mayonnaise

Wasabi mayonnaise

1/2 teaspoon wasabi paste

Instructions

1. Shred the cabbage finely with a sharp knife. This can also done with a food processer.

2. In a large skillet or large wok, heat half of the butter to fry the cabbage. It will take a while for the cabbage's to soften. However, it is important to not let it become brown.

3. Add vinegar, spices. Stir the mixture and fry for a couple of minutes. Place the chopped cabbage in a large bowl.

4. In the same saucepan, melt the butter. Add garlic, chiliflakes, and ginger. Stir fry for a few minutes.

5. Brown the ground meat. Reduce the heat.

6. Add cabbage and chopped scallions. Stir everything until hot. Salt and pepper to suit your taste. Serve with sesame oil.

7. Mix the wasabi and mayonnaise. You can start with a small amount and then add more until you achieve the desired flavor. When the stir fry is warm, add a tablespoon of wasabi mayonnaise to it.

Soup with low carbohydrate stuffed peppers
Servings: 6

Cooking time: 40 minutes

Prep Time: 10 Mins

Total Time: 50 Minutes

Ingredients

1 lb. Ground pork

1 small onion diced

1 large bell pepper diced

2 cans 14.5oz fire-roasted tomatoes

1 can 8 oz tomato sauce

1 can 14.5oz beef broth

1 bag frozen cauliflower to be thawed

Splenda: 1 tablespoon

2 cloves minced garlic

Salt and pepper to suit your tastes

Shredded cheddar or mozzarella cheese for topping

Instructions

1. Add the ground pork and onion to a large pan. Cook meat until browned and vegetables are tender. Drain the water and return to the pot.

2. Stir in the tomatoes, tomato sauce, as well as beef broth. Stir.

3. Use a blender to chop the cauliflower. Add the tomato, meat mixture to the pot.

4. Season with Splenda, garlic mince, pepper, and salt according to your taste.

5. Cover the soup and allow to simmer for 25-30 minutes on low heat.

6. Serve warm with cheddar or mozzarella cheese.

Easy Keto Pad Thai

Servings: 2

Prep Time: 15 mins

Cook Time: 8 mins

Total Time: 23 mins

Ingredients

2 tablespoons Rice wine vinegar

2 tablespoons Fish sauce

1 tablespoon Lime juice

2 large eggs

1 teaspoon Granulated artificial sweetener

2 tablespoons Peanut Oil

2 teaspoons chopped garlic

14 ounces zucchini sliced or spiralized into thin strips

5 ounces Bean sprouts

4 Scallions, chopped

2 tablespoons fresh Cilantro finely chopped

4 tablespoons chopped peanuts

Instructions

1. In a small pot, combine rice wine vinegar with fish sauce, lime juice and artificial sweetener. Boil at medium-high heat.

2. In a small bowl, beat the eggs. Add egg to boiling sauce and stir continuously. Allow eggs to cook until done. Turn off heat and let cool.

3. Place the peanut oil and garlic in a skillet. Heat on medium-high heat for approximately 1 minute. Stir in the scallions.

4. Continue to cook for one minute.

5. Spread the sauce on the zucchini, then add the bean sprouts. Allow to simmer for two minutes before removing from heat.

6. Garnish with chopped cilantro and peanuts. Serve immediately

Nutrition

Serving Size: 0.25 of Recipe

Cucumbers Caesar

Yields 2 Servings

Prep Time: 10 mins

Total time: 10 mins

Ingredients

2 medium cucumbers.

3 T Caesar Dressing

Fresh ground pepper to taste

Instructions

1. You don't even need to peel cucumbers, they are fresh from the garden.

2. Take thin slices of store-bought cukes and cut in half.

3. In a large bowl, place the sliced cucumbers. Dress liberally with Caesar Dressing.

4. Mix black pepper.

5. Enjoy your meal!

Nutrition Information:

Unsaturated Fat: 10g

SNACK RECIPES

Chicken Zucchini Poppers

Yield: 4 to 5 servings

Prep Time: 15 Minutes

Cooking time: 20 minutes

Total Time: 35 minutes

Ingredients

2 c. grated zucchini

3-4 Tablespoon cilantro, minced

1 lb. ground chicken breast (raw).

2-3 green onions, sliced

1 clove garlic, minced

1 teaspoon salt

1/2 teaspoon pepper

3/4 teaspoon cumin (optional).

Instructions

1. Mix together chicken, green onion (if you have it), zucchini, salt, garlic and cilantro in a large bowl. The mixture will be damp.

2. Take a tablespoonful or small scoop of meatballs, and mix them together. Smoothen the mixture with your hands. The size of the poppers depends on how big you make them.

To cook on the stovetop

1. On medium-low heat, heat a tablespoon of oil in the pan. Cook each side for 5-6 minutes.

2. Flip it over and continue cooking for an additional 5-10 minutes or until the centers become cooked through.

To bake:

1. Preheat oven to 400F

2. Sprinkle a few drops of avocado oil or olive oil on a parchment-lined baking sheet. Bake at 400°F for 15 to 20 minutes or until golden brown.

3. Serve with salsa or guacamole.

Parmesan Garlic Zucchini Chips

Yields: 1-3

Ingredients

1 lb (1 about 4 cups) thinly-sliced Zucchini

1 ounce finely grated Parmesan Cheese

1/8 teaspoon salt

1 finely grated minced garlic clove, or 1/8 teaspoon garlic powder

1 teaspoon apple cider vinegar

Instructions

1. Place the sliced zucchini into a medium bowl.

2. You can also add salt, Parmesan cheese and vinegar to the mixture.

3. Put on a coat.

4. Arrange slices onto dehydrator trays.

5. Dehydrate at 135° for 5-10 hours or till crispy

Healthy Baked Broccoli Tots

Prep time: 15 minutes

Cook time: 20 minutes

Total Time: 35 minutes

Calories: 26kcal

Ingredients

 2 cups or 12oz uncooked or frozen broccoli

 1 large egg

1/4 cup diced yellow onion

 1/3 cup cheddar cheese

 1/3 cup Italian breadcrumbs

 1/3 cup panko breadcrumbs

 2 Tbsp cilantro, rosemary or parsley

 1/2 tsp.

 1/2 teaspoon salt

Instructions

1. Preheat oven to 400F. Spread parchment paper on a baking tray. Put aside.

2. Boil the broccoli in boiling salted water for 1 minute. Cook for 1 minute in boiling water. Then,

drain the broccoli and shock it with a little cold tap water to stop any further cooking. Drain well.

3. Blend the eggs, cheddar, onions (or bread), seasonings, and breadcrumbs together with the chopped broccoli. You can scoop about 1.5 tbsp mix with your hands or an Ice-cream scoop. Gently press the mixture to form a tater-tot. Notice: Wash your hands after every tot to prevent them sticking to your hands.

4. Place on a lined baking tray.

5. Bake until golden brown and crisp, 18-24 minutes. Turn halfway. Enjoy hot with ranch dressing, ketchup, sriracha or ranch sauce.

Nutrition

Protein: 1g

Low Carb Cheese Crackers Recipe
Prep Time: 10 mins

Cooking time: 20 mins

Total Time: 30 mins

Servings: 30 -35

Ingredients

2 cups cheese (or any other type you prefer)

1 cup Almond Flour

2-ounce cream Cheese

1 egg

1/2 tsp sea Salt

1 tsp Rosemary (or a seasoning you choose such as chives or basil, garlic spicy chili, spicy chile, dillweed, etc.

Instructions

1. Mix the almond flour with the cream cheese in a bowl that is microwave-safe.

2. Once the almond flour and cheeses are combined, stir the ingredients together immediately. The cheese should be partially melted.

3. Allow it to cool before you add the egg. This will ensure that it doesn't get overcooked.

4. Add the sea salt, egg and seasonings of choice. You can add about 1 tablespoon to make a non

spicy mix seasoning. To make spicy seasonings, you can add 1/2 tsp.

5. Mix everything until it is well combined. Mix the cheese until it is smooth.

6. Now, place the ball made from dough on a large parchment paper. You will then place another sheet of parchment on top of it.

7. Use your rolling pin or your hands for spreading the dough into thin layers. You must ensure that your parchment paper is the same size as the baking sheet.

8. You can cut the crackers using a pizza knife into small pieces.

9. Bake each side of the crackers in a single layer at 450° for 4-6 minutes. You can bake crackers at 450 degrees for about 5 minutes. But if your dough is thicker, it may take between 6 and 9 minutes to achieve crispy cracker texture. The parchment paper makes it easy to flip the dough while it's still hot.

10. Allow crackers to cool for at least 5 minutes, then they're ready to eat.

Keto Big Mac Bites

Servings: 16

Prep time for this course: 20 minutes

Cook Time: 15 mins

Total Time: 35 mins

Ingredients

1.5 Lbs Ground Beef

1 teaspoon salt

Dill Pickle 16 slices

4 slices American Cheese

1/4 cup chopped onion

Lettuce

Sauce:

2 Tbsp yellow Mustard

1/2 cup Mayonnaise

Dill pickle relish - 4 tablespoons

1 teaspoon White wine vinegar

1 tsp Paprika

1 teaspoon Onion powder

1 tsp Garlic powder

Instructions

1. Preheat oven to 400F

2. In a large bowl, combine the onions, ground meat, and salt. Mix the ingredients until well combined.

3. Divide the beef into small, 1.5-ounce balls. You can flatten each one by pressing it down to form a mini burger patty.

4. Bake at 400F until done or for 15 minutes.

5. Once the burgers have cooked, mix all the sauce ingredients together in a bowl. Stir until well combined

6. Once the burgers have been baked, take them out of the oven and wipe off any grease.

7. Cut each cheese slice in four squares. Place one slice of cheese on each mini patty. Put the mini patty back in the oven and let it cool for a few minutes.

8. Place a few lettuce squares and a pickle piece on top of each beefball. Run a skewer along it.

9. Enjoy the sauce with the pasta.

Nutrition

Serving Size: 1 Skewer. Calories : 182kcal. Fat : 12g. Protein : 10g. Cholesterol : 36mg. Cholesterol : 36mg. Cholesterol : 414mg. Cholesterol : 36mg. Cholesterol :36mg. Cholesterol :36mg. Vitamins : 26mg. Vitamins A: 23iu. Vitamins C: 1mg.

Cauliflower Tots in Cheesy Baked

Yield: 4 Servings

Prep Time 30 Minutes

Cook Time 32 Minutes

Total Time 1 hour and 2 minutes

Ingredients

1/2 large head cauliflower coarsely chopped

1/3 cup sharp cheddar cheese

14 cup Parmesan cheese grated coarsely

2 T almond butter

1/2 teaspoon. 1/2 teaspoon.

1/2 teaspoon. Spike Seasoning and other all-purpose seasonings

Fresh-ground black Pepper to Taste

1 egg

Instructions

1. Preheat oven to 400F

2. Spray a Mini Muffin Pan, which can make 24 muffins, with non-stick spray.

3. Take out the cauliflower leaves but save the core.

4. The cauliflower should be chopped finely. Microwave the cauliflower for about 5 minutes.

5. The steam will escape if you take off the clingwrap. If there is any water left in the bowl, place the cauliflower in a colander. Let the water drain out.

www.ingramcontent.com/pod-product-compliance
Lightning Source LLC
Chambersburg PA
CBHW062139020426
42335CB00013B/1261